Navigating Mental Health in the Male Open Prison

Like the best criminological work, Schreeche-Powell's research raises much larger questions about mental health in prison, the purpose and value of punishment and the future of carceral power. It is thick with context, grounded in lived experience and unafraid to confront uncomfortable truths.

—***Professor Shadd Maruna*, Chair of Sociology, Social Policy and Criminology, University of Liverpool**

This is a compellingly rigorous study of how ostensibly progressive penal initiatives, such as peer-led induction, can solidify the 'pains of imprisonment' rather than improving prisoner well-being. Dr Schreeche-Powell' research identifies the institutional dynamics that generate and sustain manifestly deficient interventions, irrespective of their damaging consequences. This timely, deeply informed analysis of what can be done to remedy this situation should be required reading for penal policy makers.

—***Professor Eugene McLaughlin*, City St George's, University of London**

Peer support schemes have become increasingly popular in prisons and have achieved some success. Ed Schreeche-Powell's insider research offers a more critical account of peer support in open prisons. When poorly implemented in the neo-liberal prison, such schemes can become superficial tickbox exercises, used to reduce staff costs and encourage prisoner self-regulation. Schreeche-Powell reveals that to thrive, peer support schemes need proper investment and must be situated in an empowering culture.

This book will be of interest to prison staff and policymakers as well as scholars with an interest in prisons and the transformative potential of lived experience.

—***Dr Jamie Bennett*, Research associate at University of Oxford and former prison governor**

Ed Screeche-Powell speaks with a confident and convincing authority as he questions the value of peer-led induction processes in an open prison. Thoughtfully written and deeply grounded in the academic literature, the book shines a useful light on an under-studied phenomenon.

—***Emeritus Professor Nicola Padfield KC* (Hon), Emeritus Professor, University of Cambridge**

Navigating Mental Health in the Male Open Prison: Pains, Power and Peer Support

BY

ED SCHREECHE-POWELL

The University of Greenwich, UK

emerald
PUBLISHING

United Kingdom – North America – Japan – India – Malaysia – China

Emerald Publishing Limited
Emerald Publishing, Floor 5, Northspring, 21-23 Wellington Street, Leeds LS1 4DL

First edition 2026

British Library Cataloguing in Publication Data
A catalogue record for this book is available from the British Library

ISBN: 978-1-83549-707-4 (Print)
ISBN: 978-1-83549-706-7 (Online)
ISBN: 978-1-83549-708-1 (Epub)

Printed and bound by CPI Group (UK) Ltd, Croydon, CR0 4YY

INVESTOR IN PEOPLE

For Sarah; my best friend, soulmate and love, known affectionately as The Mrs, and Levi, Rhianna and Aliyah, who together make our beautiful family, alongside my mother Jaswant and sister Kathleen. As always, this work is dedicated to the memory of my late father Arthur, who never got to enjoy my academic achievements and successes.

Contents

About the Author

Ed Schreeche-Powell is a Senior Lecturer in Criminology and a programme leader in Criminology and Criminal Psychology at The University of Greenwich and an Associate Lecturer in Social and Forensic Psychology. Ed is interested in all aspects of research surrounding prisons and penal policy, with particular focus on prisoner mental health and well-being, safer custody and power-sharing initiatives in prison. Ed is also interested in the programme theory and impact evaluation of interventions in custodial settings as well as a broader interest in punitiveness within the Criminal Justice System in Western Europe. Ed is passionate in the enactment and study of lived experience to offer new criminological perspectives and is an active member of the British Convict Criminology Group. Ed also acts as an expert witness regarding prison conditions in England and Wales.

About the Author

Foreword

Every transition is a crisis. That's why we have rites of passage – to recognise and facilitate the passing of one status and the emergence of a new one. Even the smallest transition, like ending a phone call with a friend, requires a sometimes endless repetition of ritualistic goodbyes before one can finally feel safe in hanging up the receiver. Over a century ago, the folklorist and anthropologist Arnold van Gennep (1909) described the varied and elaborate rituals involved in the transition between subtle but profound life changes such as the one from childhood to adulthood, from singledom to marriage or from student to graduate. He argued that all of these transitions were not just facilitated, but indeed made possible, through what he termed 'rites of passage' involving a famous tripartite structure of separation, liminality and incorporation (see Turner, 1967).

The experience of punishment in the criminal justice system is replete with enormous transitions (hence crises) of this sort, including the well-known traumas of moving from society into custody (separation) and from custody back into society (incorporation). The pains of these transitions are well recognised and widely studied (see Maruna, 2011a), and indeed the prison may be the best known 'liminal space' in contemporary anthropological enquiry. Yet, far less research has examined the equally profound and surely traumatic transition from 'closed' prison conditions to an 'open' prison, which Schreeche-Powell has chosen for the research site of this incredibly important study. As major life transitions go, this transition into open prison conditions (which Schreeche-Powell calls a 'double liminality' somewhere between incarceration and freedom) is surely among the most daunting and difficult – far more so than ending a phone call. Yet (perhaps partially because the lack of previous research attention to this process) prison management and staff have heretofore invested relatively little attention to addressing this crisis through facilitating structured rites of passage.

In this sense, the development of the peer support scheme described in this book is anthropologically insightful in this regard and, in my opinion, is something to be commended. After all, the primary challenge of the transition is leaving the familiar for the unknown. How can a person be expected to navigate a change into the unknown, when, by definition, they have never experienced it, do not know what is coming or how to navigate it? The only solution to this is to identify those who have walked the path and to use them as a guide. Want to transition from being a plumber to being an academic? You need to find a PhD supervisor who has already been on the journey to act as a mentor for your training. Want to transition from being an academic to a plumber? You need to identify a master craftsman with whom you can arrange an apprenticeship while you learn the ropes. So, as in every other field, the designation of more experienced peers to act as mentors for those transitioning to open prison conditions is on its face the right idea for the right challenge. It is also, nicely, in synch with the growing movement around the value of capitalising on 'lived experience' that has spread from the worlds of addiction recovery and mental health into the prisons world, ever so reluctantly, in the past decade.

Unfortunately, as Schreeche-Powell illustrates in rich anthropological detail here, the prison system in England and Wales is going through a different kind of crisis, as an entire service. Massively over-crowded, starved of resources and losing the most experienced and dedicated staff to better jobs, HM Prison Service has entered what appears to be a permanent state of crisis. Perhaps the lowest point in the system's history, the system-wide lockdown during the COVID-19 crisis (see Maruna et al., 2022) still reverberates throughout the system today as manifested in record levels of violence, self-harm, suicidality and distress among those inside.

As is so often the case in such dire circumstances, the best of intentions (like those motivating the creation of the peer support scheme) have led not just to weak results but, Schreeche-Powell finds, have actually been counter-productive, making a difficult process even worse. That is, the cure appears worse than the disease. Peer support volunteers feel like their labour is being exploited 'on the cheap' with the shifting of the burden of responsibility from over-stretched and poorly paid (but still paid!) prison staff to their backs. Meanwhile, those making the transition are more abandoned than ever as a result of staff resistance and undermining of the scheme, entrenched managerialism and punitive penal cultures inside the institutions. By asking peer support volunteers to legitimise and even shoulder the blame for such regimes, Schreeche-Powell argues, the peer support scheme clearly serves institutional interests but may create more stress for those in custody. This 'peer support paradox' – where an intervention meant to mitigate the pains of imprisonment appears to have created additional pains – may represent yet another transition in the nature of penal power in a new era of low budget quick fixes. It also represents a stark cautionary tale for those of us, like Schreeche-Powell himself, who are instinctively in support of efforts like this to empower mutual aid among those in prison.

In short, this modest-appearing case study turns out to be about a great deal more than just an assessment of a peer support scheme. Like the best criminological work, Schreeche-Powell's research raises much larger questions about mental health in prison, the purpose and value of punishment and the future of carceral power. Partially, this is due to the rich and thick fieldwork methodology. As argued in the book's conclusion, real evidence-led policy thinking needs to transcend short-term evaluation research (as important as such work is) and include rich ethnographic and qualitative research like that featured in this study. Whereas evaluation research encourages quick-fix 'intervention-itis' like the momentum behind the peer support scheme, this in-depth analysis provides a much more thoughtful and nuanced guide for understanding why even good ideas seem to go so routinely wrong.

Mostly, however, this book's rich insights might themselves be understood as resulting from Schreeche-Powell's own lived experience of the criminal legal system, discussed insightfully and instructively in this book's outstanding methodological chapter ('Researching Lived Experience with Lived Experience'). The field of criminology is going through something of an identity crisis of its own at the moment with the rise and rise of the lived experience movement and the struggle for epistemic justice challenging the authority of traditional academic research to speak 'on behalf' of those in prison (see e.g., Darley et al., 2023; Earle et al., 2023). Like every transition, this one has already proven to be a bit of a bumpy ride with pushback and resistance from both sides and in-fighting even among the lived experience community. Fortunately, the field now has a number of wise mentors like Schreeche-Powell, who have both *academic* and *lived* expertise, and can therefore guide us through this transition to a future of knowledge equity in the field. Consider this outstanding book to be a small but crucial step on that journey.

Professor Shadd Maruna
Chair of Sociology, Social Policy and Criminology
University of Liverpool

Acknowledgements

I thank all who have been part of the journey so far; there are too many to name. That said, I want to give special thanks to Professor Caroline Chatwin and Professor Marisa Silvestri. You have played many roles in my journey as first my educators, then colleagues but most important is our friendship.

Big thanks are also reserved for Dr Rod Earle, Dr Atalanta Goulandris as well as my colleagues and friends at The University of Greenwich and formerly The University of Kent. Thank you for all the support, guidance and opportunities. Thank you to those who gave their time to be sounding boards for my ideas and narratives (of all varieties), read passages and give feedback and also to those who kindly endorsed my work.

Special thanks to my friends who have stood by me and supported me over the years – particularly Kym and Kim.

I am truly blessed to do the things I love for the people I love, and in doing so, I hope that I make a difference to the lives of those imprisoned.

Chapter 1

Introduction

> Prisons, like prostitutes, have always been with us but, over time and place have changed radically in conditions, attributes and functions as well as in their name, character and rationale. (Potter, 2019)

The constant flux within prisons is intrinsic to the pain that prisoners experience while confined within the walls of our penal institutions. Make no mistake about it, pain is experienced by each and every individual imprisoned, regardless of the underpinning philosophy of punishment and purpose of imprisonment. The delivery of pain is synonymous with punishment and imprisonment and has been an enduring theme in the study of prisons.

> Whilst most inmates, including long-term prisoners, adjust successfully to prison life, many do not cope well with the pains of imprisonment. Maladaptive responses such as emotional disorders, self-mutilation, suicide attempts, and prison misbehaviour are most common during the early phases of induction. (Adams, 1992, p. 27)

While many imprisoned are admitted initially from the court, others are later received through prison transfer, which itself is a minefield. The most common reasons for transfer are changes in security category and sentence progression. Prisoners may transfer so that they can, for example, take part in an offending behaviour course in another prison, a course that might help to reduce their risk level. Some prisoners, in the final weeks of their sentence, move to a prison closer to home to support their resettlement or 'local discharge'. Ideally, this gives someone the opportunity to make links for resettlement and coordinate their release with their family and external offender manager. Other reasons include prison staff concerns about prisoner safety or perceived vulnerability to other prisoners, as well as consideration of medical and disability needs, but many will have received status allowing them to move to a lower security category prison due to their progress and to further their progress through the system.

Navigating Mental Health in the Male Open Prison, 1–15

Published under exclusive licence by Emerald Publishing Limited
doi:10.1108/978-1-83549-706-720251001

Transfer from closed prison to open prison is a core element of this book. Transfers between establishments are a staple of prison life in England and Wales. Between July and September 2024, there were 23,818 incidences of prisoner transfer, with 20,398 prisoners having at least one incidence of transfer. Both figures represent increases of 8% since the same period of 2023 with 8%–10% of such transfers to Category D – open prisons (Ministry of Justice, 2025a). For prisoners, transfer is a tough and psychologically taxing prospect, underpinned by the lurking the *fear of the unknown* alongside the claustrophobia and physical anguish of the journey on the 'sweat bus' (the term 'cattle class' is never more apt than when discussing prison transport). Then, to arrive at a new establishment and be plunged further into a chasm of unknowing during the arrival and transition period is an apparent and very real concern. At a time where a tailored package of support, care and information should be provided, there are glaring deficiencies. How do I know this? Ethnographic pioneer Bronislaw Malinowski has said 'in order to explain a cultural product it is necessary to know it. And to know it, in matters of thought and emotion, is to have experienced it' (cited in Earle, 2016, p. 1). I have lived it, endured it and witnessed it on numerous occasions during my own experience of imprisonment, before researching it.

Such experiences culminate in immense distress and evidence the 'corrosive and demanding nature of imprisonment' (Liebling, 1999, p. 286). This exposes what Giddens (1984) describes as a state of 'ontological insecurity' that can swamp an individual's psychological coping mechanisms. Around 1 in 4 adults are diagnosed with a mental health illness during their lifespan, and many more will be subject to changes in their mental health and well-being, with prisoners more likely to suffer from such problems than those in general population outside of prison. Vast amounts of the prisoner population have mental health problems, with the potential for their issues to be exacerbated by imprisonment (Adatia, 2010; Fazel & Danesh, 2002; Singleton et al., 1998; Stewart, 2008). Recently, there has been a renewed vigour in the public domain for addressing mental health with its widespread recognition as a public health issue worldwide raising its profile and agenda. Public attitudes have continued to align with a picture of greater tolerance, awareness and recognition of mental health issues with support for treatment rather than punishment of underlying problems (Esmée Fairbairn Foundation, 2004). The Joint Committee on Human Rights investigation (2004) into deaths in custody recommended prioritising the reduction of self-inflicted deaths and self-harm, alongside improving pre-reception, reception and induction areas which are identified as critical stressors of mental health issues.

The Safer Custody Group was established in 2001 to deliver a strategy across prisons in England and Wales with the following aims: to move from awareness to protection, to invest more resources where the risks are highest, to provide a better physical environment for prisoners (especially upon reception), to provide more training to frontline staff relating to mental health and suicide prevention, to develop better self-harm interventions, to increase peer listeners and to develop better inter-disciplinary relations. It also recognised that reducing the number of prisoners held as 'imperative' could improve mental health outcomes relating to family ties, social exclusion, staffing and resource pressure, regarding instability and constraint (Sedenu, 2005).

One strategy employed by the Safer Custody Group, both to meet safer custody aims and to mitigate the pain associated with imprisonment, was to introduce the use of prisoner peer support workers to support prisoners through a variety of interventions across the prison estate. Peer-led induction is one such intervention that utilises peer support workers alongside staff as a power-sharing initiative to deliver support and information, advice and guidance, specifically to prisoners entering a penal establishment. Every prisoner arriving at a prison will encounter some form of induction and will be mandated to engage with it although some prisoners may refuse or be resistant. Peer-led induction is an intervention that is adaptable to different prison establishments with differing facilities and populations. Its roots, however, can be firmly positioned among the core tenets of the Induction Insiders Scheme which it adopts. The Insiders Scheme states aims to improve the quality of life for prisoners by promoting community responsibility, supportive relationships and a caring environment. It does so by empowering and training prisoners to collaborate in the reception and induction process so that they might establish supportive relationships, offer reassurance and disseminate relevant and accurate information about the prison and its regime (HMP Safer Custody Group, 2005). Peer support workers also provide additional support to first time and/or vulnerable prisoners, help with basic needs (letter writing, filling out forms and applications), identify gaps in literature that prisoners need, alert staff of any concerns about any new prisoner including about those at risk of self-harm, suicide or bullying, record initial contact and referrals and follow up with prisoners where required.

Blagden and Perrin (2014, p. 17) advance that 'peer support schemes have existed in prisons for decades yet have only recently garnered attention (…) regarding how prisons can better support their inhabitants'. This is little narrow, however, as it neglects a host of other reasons for their rationale, such as institutional benefits in the face of an increasingly austere prison system characterised by low staffing levels, managerialism, poor resourcing as well as high rates of suicide and self-harm. However, as Maruna (2011a) cautions, '[i]t's not an unfamiliar habit to dress up failed old policy as a seemingly new exciting paradigm shift by simply changing a few buzz words' (p. 7).

With the implementation of peer support interventions across the prison estate gathering momentum, there remains about them a conspicuous absence of evaluative study and literature and as to whether they are delivering their intended outcomes (Perrin, 2024; Schreeche-Powell, 2020). The assertion by Maruna (2011a, p. 8) that 'practices seem to be operating in a vacuum, with no clear explanation for the process is supposed to work' can be extended to prison interventions, and this is especially true to those surrounding peer-led induction. This is in part because research to date on reception into custody and adaptation largely focuses on the early days of custody following reception into prison from the court after sentence. As such, it has neglected the experience of inter-prison transfer from closed prisons and reception and adaptation to a new establishment. The latter shares many experiential factors with the former and also introduces the prisoner to a range of differing dynamics that interact with the process of, and contribute to, the 'tightness' of their penal experience. Whereas in closed establishments prisoners are subject to a more structured regime that is built on routine, prescriptiveness and dependence on prison staff (Statham et al., 2021; Sykes, 1958), it is much the opposite in the open estate. This transition is fraught with difficulties and challenges, which requires psychological adaptation to navigate and survive.

To fit into the prison world in which they live in, prisoners must learn both the formal and informal governing guidelines (Weinrath, 2016). While they improve their capacity for living in constrained environments, they deteriorate in terms of their ability to live independently in the community (Berger & Luckman, 1967; Clemmer, 1940; Honeywell, 2015). Some scholars have suggested that prisoners serving long-term sentences fail to make judgements for themselves, since these adaptations become increasingly deep-rooted the longer the sentence (Cohen & Taylor, 1981). The England and Wales prison system's Category D open establishments have the lowest level of security and are designed to reduce some of the negative effects of incarceration by giving inmates more freedom and autonomy (Crewe, 2011a; Shammas, 2014, 2017). However, as HM Inspectorate of Prisons (2021) caution:

> ...prisoners in open prisons have consistently told [...] how nervous they are about the future. They have become so used to the predictable routines of prison life that they have lost everyday skills, such as negotiating transport or using a smartphone. They are often uncertain where they will live, how relationships will have changed with their children and families, and what they will do for work.

Given these concerns, the use of peer-led induction serves a crucial function in the open prison to support adaptation and transition at this time of great stress and anxiety. Yet, prisons have long been sites of power, discipline and control, where governance mechanisms evolve in response to shifting penal philosophies and institutional demands. While traditional forms of coercion – physical confinement, deprivation and overt disciplinary measures – have been central to imprisonment, contemporary penal regimes increasingly rely on managerialism and responsibilisation as mechanisms of governance. Managerialism, with its emphasis on efficiency, cost-effectiveness and performance metrics, has restructured prison operations, prioritising bureaucratic compliance over meaningful rehabilitation. At the same time, responsibilisation has emerged as a strategy that transfers the burden of rehabilitation and self-governance onto prisoners themselves, often masking institutional disengagement under the guise of autonomy and empowerment. This book critically engages with these interwoven themes, demonstrating how penal power is no longer exercised solely through coercion but through the strategic delegation of responsibility, the outsourcing of adaptation processes to prisoners and the pervasive influence of managerial priorities on intervention design and delivery.

The Study

The study upon which this book is based (Schreeche-Powell, 2023) has harnessed the authors lived experience, recognising that transfer, transition and adaptation to open prison as a time of great uncertainty, insecurity and anxiety. It questions the impact that the frontline intervention of peer-led induction has on a prisoner's experience of imprisonment. In doing so, it draws upon qualitative interviews with ex-prisoners who have experienced peer-led induction in the open prison estate and prison officers involved in the delivery of peer-led induction. This study explored the impact of these early days of transition and adaptation in open prison, following the critical process of transfer, on the mental health and well-being of prisoners and the extent to which peer-led induction alleviates this, or not. In doing so, it:

- identified the challenges and difficulties experienced by males who are imprisoned at the 'critical time' of the transfer process, the early days of custody in open prisons post-transfer and their impact on their mental health and well-being;
- explored the experience of current peer-led induction initiatives on the mental health and well-being of males who are imprisoned in open prisons;
- developed a theoretical informed analysis of the 'peer-led induction model' as a power-sharing initiative between staff and males who are imprisoned;
- explored the nature and motivations of the peer-led induction as a power-sharing initiative and its impact upon the legitimacy of the custodial regime and setting from the perspective of people who are imprisoned.

The central questions that the study answered to achieve these aims and objectives are:

- What is the impact of peer-led induction upon the mental health and well-being of people who are imprisoned in open prisons in the early transitional days of custody following transfer?
- How does the re-configuration of penal power through power-sharing initiatives manifest in the experience of transfer and imprisonment of people who are imprisoned?
- In what ways and to what extent do power-sharing initiatives impact the 'tightness' of imprisonment?

It therefore allows the book to consider peer-led induction through the theoretical lens of power and pain and as such, how peer-led induction as a power-sharing initiative interacts with 'tightness' in the experience of imprisonment at these crucial times.

Why Study Men?

Approximately, 50% of men arriving in custody being at risk of anxiety and depression and 15% of males reporting symptoms of psychosis while in custody.

It is further reported that nearly one in five of those diagnosed with a mental health issue or concern received no care or support from a mental health professional while in prison (Prison Reform Trust, 2019a). Furthermore, 16% of men imprisoned in England and Wales had received community mental health treatment in the year prior to custody (Durcan, 2008; Fazel & Danesh, 2002; Fraser, 2009; Jewkes, 2007; National Audit Office, 2017; Peay, 2017; Singleton et al., 1998). Self-harm is an issue of central interest, especially as it is often the manifestation of mental health issues that prisoners experience, and its measure contributes to literature surrounding the extent of mental health issues in prisons. The existing evidence based on self-harm is complex and often subsumed by studies focusing on suicide. It also tends not to clearly separate men and women.

This foundation provides one primary motivation underpinning the use of a solely male prisoner sample in this study. As such, there is still much to learn about the motivations for self-harm in prisons, the risk factors for future self-harm and suicide and how these might differ for men and women, given what has been described as an 'explosion of male self-injury in groups who might be considered socially disadvantaged. . .adults in prisons' (Adler & Adler, 2011, p. 20). This is particularly true for self-harm by adult men.

What we do know, however, from the paucity of evidence is that there are indications of a range of intrapersonal and interpersonal reasons underpinning such behaviours. Gardner et al. (2016) in their study into the reasons for non-suicidal self-harm in adult male offenders saw 82.9% of the sample endorse a reason that was intrapersonal in nature, and 72.5% endorse interpersonal. Intrapersonal reasons frequently identified were releasing emotional pressure, reducing anxiety, frustration and anger, punishing themselves, reacting to feeling unhappy. Notably, the seriousness of self-harm is more pronounced in males than females while the rate of self-inflicted deaths in males is more elevated than in females (MOJ, 2025a). This resonates with an earlier study by Hawton et al. (2014), who found in their analysis of self-harm in the England and Wales prison estate that 10% of instances in males were of medium or high lethality compared with 3% in females, illustrating the gendered ways of self-injuring (Adler & Adler, 2011), with women also displaying a tendency to make smaller cuts and men more inclined to make more substantial, deeper cuts and burns.

It can be argued that characteristics of the masculine identity of the male prison population are a central issue which has served to underpin this lack of knowledge, as well as providing some explanation for the mental health, self-harm and suicide issues across the prison estate among the male prison population. Kupers (2005) highlights an intensification of gender dynamic in prison settings. There is an expression of a toxic masculinity, which is socially destructive. These toxic hegemonic characteristics tend to proliferate wildly in prison settings (Kupers, 2005) and are often the measurement yardstick against which male prisoners, and men in totality, are measured, either by others or themselves. According to Kupers (2005), in prison settings the rules of this masculinity comprise a real man or stand-up con who: (i) does not display weakness, (ii) does not display emotions other than anger, (iii) does not depend on anyone, (iv) is never vulnerable, (v) does not snitch, (vi) does not cooperate with the authorities and (vii) suffers pain in silence.

This 'mask' of traditional masculinity that imprisoned men put on in prison often hides an emotional struggle. These characteristics in their totality are an unreasonable endeavour for any man, yet that does not prevent males 'trying, valiantly and vainly to measure up' (Kimmel, 1994, p. 272). The failure to do so through an inability to embody these rules is affirmation of the rules' power. Achieving the rules is often ascribed as the reasoning for a man's confusion and pain. The fear of failing is arguably illustrated by a lack of male willingness to talk and to identify mental health and well-being deficiencies they are experiencing. Quite simply, masculine characteristics restrict men from having emotional responses or, at the very least, articulating them in the public domain. It is widely situated that males, especially male prisoners, are predisposed to difficulties communicating their thoughts, feelings and emotions. Male prisoners who are actively aligned with masculine gender role orientations are significantly less likely to express any interest in seeking psychological help than other individuals with, for example, a female gender orientation or restrictive emotional characteristics of males (Good et al., 1989; Nam et al., 2010). These men experience difficulties in adulthood in experiencing, accurately expressing and responding effectively to their own emotions (Addis, 2011; Green & Addis, 2012; Green & Jakupcak, 2016). The toxic masculinity that pervades penal institutions makes seeking help even more difficult. Prisoners' 'survival behaviours' while navigating the brutal mechanisms of custody and the 'lags code' mean that they play their cards close to their chest, refusing to reveal their vulnerabilities. As such, they do not seek help and the problems magnify. Fear of stigmatisation is a prevalent and dominating consideration for the male prisoner.

In this vein, Whitlock et al. (2011) found that healthcare professionals are less likely to assess males for non-suicidal self-harm because of their perception and identification of men as being associated with or being the embodiment of hegemonic masculinity. There is an expectation from professionals that men will externalise their emotions rather than internalise them, as associated with female emotion or because of the generational, structural or societal normalisation of gender differences in the specific types of self-harming behaviours (for example, 'boys will be boys'). This often means that at a structural and organisational level within the prison institution and within healthcare provision, both prison and clinical personnel responses are 'missing' mental health, self-harm and suicidality issues in males.

Stearns (1979, p. 1) observes that the complexity surrounding masculinity means that 'the only common currency is a sense that masculinity is sorely troubled in modern society, both in concept and practice'. What is apparent from current literature surrounding the masculine identity of male prisoners is that the traditional conceptualisations of hegemonic masculinity and contemporary conceptualisations of the masculine identity transcend across one another, and while some aspects of these identities are salient, others are more prominently dependent on social context. All add to the ongoing debates and intrigue into the male prisoner, illuminating the gaps in, and need for more empirical literature, especially concerning mental health.

Why Study Transfer and Transition to Open Prison?

There are currently 107 male prisons in the England and Wales across the differing security categories (Table 1), with 23, 571 prison officers (Bands 3–5) and 5,592 full-time equivalent Band 2 operational support staff in post employed (HMPPS, 2025). Only a small proportion of these are prisons are local, as in they receive individuals directly from the court following charges for an offence. Yet there is a disproportionate focus on the early days in custody of those entering these prisons and a lack of focus on the many other prisons receiving prisoners through inter-prison transfer, given that these prison transfers are a frequent event. Between July and September 2024, there were 23,818 incidences of prisoner transfer, with 20,398 prisoners having at least one incidence of transfer (MOJ, 2025a). By granting offenders more freedom and autonomy, the Category D open prison facilities of the England and Wales prison system, which have the lowest level of security, are intended to lessen some of the negative impacts of incarceration. Many

Table 1. Prison Security Classifications.

Prison Type	Category	Prison Description
Closed prison	A (High Security)	Those whose escape would be highly dangerous to the public or national security. Offences that may result in consideration for Category A or Restricted Status include: (Attempted) murder, rape, indecent assault, robbery or conspiracy to rob (with firearms), firearms offences, importing or supplying Class A controlled drugs, possessing or supplying explosives, offences connected with terrorism.
	B	Those who pose a risk to the public but may not require maximum security, but for whom escape still needs to be made very difficult.
	C	Those who cannot be trusted in open conditions but who are unlikely to try to escape.
Open prison	D	Those who can be reasonably trusted not to try to escape, and are given the privilege of an open prison. Prisoners at 'D Cat'. (as it is commonly known) prisons, are, subject to approval, given release on temporary licence (ROTL) to work in the community or to go on 'home leave'.

Source: MOJ (n.d.).

who are housed in these 13 open prisons must already be deemed low risk to the public and of absconding prior to accessing open conditions (Statham et al., 2021). Achieving Category D status as a prisoner and gaining a place at an open prison is a result of good conduct, engaging with sentence planning targets and having positive relations with prison staff (Meško & Hacin, 2018).

Conditions in Category D prisons are designed to be aligned with that of the outside world to allow those men who are imprisoned to adjust and acculturate towards regaining independence and day-to-day functioning outside of the walls (Statham et al., 2021). Release on temporary licence (ROTL) is a key provision allowing prisoner release to undertake employment, education, medical appointments and home visits with family (Danks & Bradley, 2018; Statham et al., 2021). The dynamic of a lower security setting with less staffing and security measures means that there is a higher threshold of responsibility behaviourally for prisoners. Statham et al. (2021, p. 5) state that further understanding is needed to clarify the ways in which open establishments support prisoner reintegration as 'whilst release is often eagerly anticipated, individuals face numerous barriers as they leave a place of familiar routine to enter more unpredictable circumstances'. However, this is also true when leaving closed conditions for open ones.

Prisoners' status is also precarious, and a number of psychological manifestations can result from concerns surrounding prisoners being returned to closed conditions from open establishments for reasons such as substance misuse, feeling threatened and bullied, or a use of violence (Statham et al., 2021). There can be the notion of 'too much too soon' and the pressure, after years of penal dependence, of suddenly having to be responsible for a variety of different roles between family, employment and prison life. As Honeywell (2015) explores, this can be overwhelming for the individual. Prisoner misconduct is seen as stemming from an individual's unsuccessful adaptation to life in the Category D prison and the inability to grasp the basic elements of the prisoner subculture (Meško & Hacin, 2018).

In an open setting where there are new norms and a sense of independence, the internalised expectations, regulations and adjustments developed in closed settings are likely to be inapplicable. People's personal resources are put under pressure when there are no physical boundaries, which can be unsettling for people who have grown reliant on others (Crewe, 2011b). Constrained freedom then becomes the source of experienced pain, described by Shammas (2014, p. 104) as the 'pains of freedom where freedom can be experienced as ambiguous, bittersweet or tainted'. As Statham et al. (2021, p. 731) articulate, 'open establishments are not always the coveted institutions they're expected to be, and the precise coping mechanisms adopted by individuals who successfully remain within these conditions are unknown ingenuity'. Despite the open prison being a key institution for individuals who are transitioning, 'extremely little research has been conducted within it', (Statham et al., 2021, p. 730) highlighting that it lags behind the rapidly developing body of literature relating to the closed prison environment, with empirical research on the experiences of those within the open prison limited (Marder et al., 2021; Mjåland et al., 2023).

This book is essential and timely because prisons remain in a state of crisis, with mental health concerns at the forefront of institutional failings. Despite decades of reform efforts, self-harm, suicidality and psychological distress among prisoners continue to escalate, exposing the systemic inability of penal institutions to provide meaningful support. Austerity-driven cutbacks, implemented in English prisons by the 2012 Benchmarking Programme, led to a dramatic reduction in the prison workforce and budgetary constraints, with prisons further unable to provide safe environments for rising prison populations (Ismail, 2020, 2022). In the wake of this melting pot of issues, focus on mental health and support made its way back onto the frontline of policy agenda, with increasing reliance on peer-led interventions emerging as a strategy to address them. Around 7% of prisoners in England and Wales are documented as participating as peer supporters (South et al., 2014), reflecting the growing institutional reliance on peer-led initiatives to address systemic gaps in mental health and well-being provision, yet despite this increasing prevalence of peer interventions in the prison system, comprehensive academic studies on their mechanisms, effectiveness and limitations remain relatively scarce and underexplored in academic research.

This book addresses a critical gap in the literature, examining how peer-led induction operates within open prisons, how power is reconfigured through responsibilisation strategies and whether these interventions genuinely support prisoner well-being or merely extend institutional control in more insidious ways. As prisons continue to struggle with the mental health crisis, staff shortages, overcrowding and resource limitations, understanding the lived realities of peer interventions, their structural limitations and their potential for both support and harm is more urgent than ever. One of the central arguments of this book is that penal interventions, when not carefully designed and evaluated, can produce unintended harm rather than alleviating distress. Drawing on the concept of iatrogenesis – originally used in medicine to describe harm caused by treatment – this book applies the concept to prison governance, demonstrating how peer-led induction, instead of supporting prisoner adaptation, often intensifies psychological distress, responsibilisation pressures and institutional tightness. By interrogating the intersection of peer support, mental health and penal power, this research challenges assumptions about the progressive nature of interventions and asks whether prisons and their mechanisms can ever truly function as supportive spaces conducive with positive mental health outcomes for those at 'stressor' points of imprisonment.

Structure

Chapter 2 critically examines the enduring failures of penal reform in addressing the mental health crisis in prisons, demonstrating how penal power remains the defining force within prison institutions despite over a century of reform efforts. By tracing key historical reports – including the Gladstone Committee (1895), English Prisons Today (1922), the Woolf Report (1991) and the Bradley Report (2009) – it reveals how reformist discourse has repeatedly recognised the need for change, yet systemic suffering has persisted, with control consistently prioritised over care reinforcing systemic suffering rather than alleviating it. This sustained failure underpins what Allison (2017) asserts as a 'mental health crisis' across the prison estate in England and Wales.

At the heart of this analysis is the reconfiguration of penal power. The chapter explores the transition from 'hard to soft power', where compliance is enforced through psychological governance, responsibilisation and perpetual risk assessment. Drawing on Sykes' (1958) 'pains of imprisonment' and Crewe's (2011a, 2011b) contemporary pains and concept of 'tightness', it argues that contemporary penal regimes have not reduced suffering but instead introduced new pains embedded within mechanisms that claim to support. These pains – characterised by uncertainty, the burden of self-governance and the erosion of personal agency – are particularly pronounced in open prisons, where autonomy is illusory, and the demand for self-regulation exacerbates psychological distress. By considering the experiences of prisoners transitioning between institutions, this chapter introduces additional and forgotten 'pains of imprisonment' linked to adaptation. These transition-specific pains reinforce how penal power operates through instability, ensuring that suffering remains central to the penal experience, even in supposedly progressive regimes. The chapter argues that despite repeated policy interventions, imprisonment remains a system of 'legitimated pain delivery' (Carlen, 1994), where psychological suffering is structurally embedded.

Chapter 3 explores how prisons, under resource constraints, have adopted a 'doing more with less' approach, which in part positions peer interventions as a cost-effective response to the persistent challenges of prisoner adaptation and psychological distress. Peer supporters are used as intermediaries between staff and prisoners, legitimising official communication and improving engagement with institutional processes. Their lived experience enhances credibility and relatability, making them more effective in influencing prisoner behaviour and alleviating distress than prison staff alone. However, while these interventions are framed as beneficial, they also serve institutional interests by transferring aspects of prison governance onto prisoners themselves, reinforcing responsibilisation. The chapter outlines the primary typologies of peer support situating peer support within a broader theoretical framework, drawing on Social Learning Theory, Social Inoculation Theory and Differential Association Theory to examine how prisoners influence one another's adaptation and engagement with institutional structures. Central to this discussion is the 'buffering effect', wherein peer support mitigates some of the psychological burdens of imprisonment, particularly for those undergoing prison transition and adaptation. However, while often presented as beneficial for both individuals and institutions, the chapter critically examines the fragile underbelly – where peer support schemes can be manipulated, co-opted by the institution or inadvertently reinforce hierarchies of power and exclusion. Ultimately, this chapter interrogates whether peer-led initiatives serve as genuine mechanisms of support or function as another extension of penal control, responsibilisation and institutional cost-cutting.

Chapter 4 critically reflects on the methodological journey of researching lived experience with lived experience. It examines the challenges, adaptations and ethical complexities of conducting qualitative research with a 'hard-to-reach' population – both prisoners and prison officers – while navigating the researcher's own positionality as a former prisoner. Drawing on Merton's (1972) 'Insider Doctrine', the chapter explores how the researcher occupies both insider and outsider statuses. In doing so, it considers the liminality of this space and the performativity of the betwixt and between, moving fluidly between roles depending on the research context. It considers the implications of this positionality on data collection, access and rapport-building, particularly in relation to recruitment challenges and the role of gatekeepers in facilitating engagement with prison officers.

The chapter also details the methodological adaptations necessitated by the COVID-19 pandemic, which led to a shift from away immersive ethnographic research to research with 'ethnographic edges' (Davies, 2015), emphasising the importance of methodological flexibility in criminology. To navigate the emotional and ethical complexities of researching a shared experience, the chapter considers a reflexive framework, examining five interrelated themes: self-disclosure, rapport, reciprocity, emotional labour and ethical dilemmas. Through this lens, the chapter explores the tensions of researcher identity, the responsibilities of amplifying participant voices and the 'ethical hangovers' associated with fieldwork. Ultimately, the chapter argues that lived experience research is a dynamic and relational act, requiring deep reflexivity, ethical sensitivity and a commitment to methodological adaptability in order to balance empathy, objectivity and a commitment to acknowledging the complexities of insider/outsider positionality in the research process.

Chapter 5 examines the structural and institutional constraints that disrupt the effectiveness of peer-led induction in open prisons, focusing on how prison culture, staff resistance and managerialism shape the delivery of peer support interventions. Using prisoner mentee and prison staff perspectives, it interrogates the role of both peer support workers and prison staff in the facilitation of these schemes, questioning whether they function as genuine support mechanisms or are compromised by competing institutional priorities. Applying 'Knowledge Management' and 'Knowledge Sharing' frameworks within a penal context, the chapter explores how knowledge is transferred, withheld and controlled in prison environments, where access to information is deeply intertwined with power hierarchies and institutional logics. It highlights how the strategic withholding and filtering of knowledge by both prison staff and peer support workers reinforces a bureaucratic 'tick-box culture' and limits the transformative potential of peer interventions. It considers how the strain of transfer and adaptation compounds mental distress, positioning prison transition as a critical moment of vulnerability. Expanding on Sykes' (1958) and Crewe's (2011a, 2011b) work, the chapter introduces the concept of 'double liminality' where prisoners exist in an ambiguous state of transition compounding their psychological distress. It reveals how staff resistance, ineffective leadership and tensions surrounding power-sharing undermine peer-led induction, resulting in a managerialist approach that prioritises bureaucratic compliance over prisoner well-being. While pockets of good practice exist, systemic failures, institutional inertia and entrenched penal governance structures hinder the potential for meaningful peer intervention. The chapter challenges the assumption that peer-led schemes are inherently progressive, arguing that until structural and cultural barriers are addressed, peer-led induction will remain an exercise in bureaucratic formalism rather than a substantive tool for prisoner adaptation and support.

Chapter 6 critically examines responsibilisation as a dominant strategy in contemporary penal practice, particularly within peer-led interventions in open prisons. Responsibilisation, which revolves around self-governance and self-regulation, is widely framed as a means of empowering prisoners to take control of their own rehabilitation and adaptation to custody. However, this chapter interrogates the reality of responsibilisation in practice, revealing it as a strategy that masks institutional disengagement, weakens formal support structures and exacerbates the mental health and well-being challenges faced by prisoners. Rather than fostering autonomy, responsibilisation often transfers the burden of adaptation onto prisoners themselves, operating under the illusion of agency while failing to deliver a genuinely needs-driven approach to induction. The chapter explores how responsibilisation interacts with the concept of 'tightness', capturing the stress, uncertainty and anxiety experienced by prisoners as they navigate transfer, transition and adaptation to open conditions. It reveals how prison staff and peer support workers often lack visibility and engagement in the process, leaving new inductees to navigate adaptation with minimal guidance. This absence of structured support compounds psychological distress, reinforcing a culture of institutional neglect where peer interventions serve managerial, rather than prisoner-focused, outcomes. Further, it highlights how self-regulation is framed as a mechanism, ensuring compliance while allowing staff to justify disengagement and peer support workers to act in self-interest. The chapter argues that while responsibilisation is discursively framed as a progressive and empowering strategy, in reality, it functions to deepen prisoner stress and undermines the effectiveness of peer-led induction.

Chapter 7 advances conceptualisations of the unintended consequences of peer-led interventions, framing them as 'iatrogenic' outcomes – where interventions designed to support adaptation in fact exacerbate harm. It situates the prison as a site of 'Institutional Pain Delivery', where peer support schemes, rather than alleviating distress, often reinforce the structural inequalities and penal governance strategies that sustain prisoner suffering. Through analysis of managerial, staff and mentor motivations, the chapter reveals how peer-led induction has been co-opted as a tool for institutional efficiency and means rather than a needs-driven intervention. This reflects the saturation of peer interventions across the prison estate as quick fixes that serve managerial interests rather than genuinely addressing prisoner well-being. These schemes lack the informed theoretical and evaluative grounding necessary to ensure their effectiveness, operating without a clear programme theory or structured evaluation framework. The absence of rigorous oversight has created a vacuum where interventions are assumed to be beneficial despite growing evidence that they produce unintended harms. This chapter introduces the concept of intervention iatrogenesis, drawing on Illich (1975, 1976) and Cohen (1988, 1998) to examine how peer interventions generate new pains of imprisonment rather than mitigating them. It argues that institutional belligerence – marked by reactive, poorly structured policy implementation symbolic of 'intervention-it is' – has led to expansion of peer-led schemes without the necessary evaluative mechanisms to determine their efficacy. This results in a 'peer support paradox', where initiatives designed to offer support are instead instrumentalised as mechanisms of coercion, responsibilisation and control.

The chapter engages with managerialism as a key driver of these unintended outcomes, situating its discussion within broader critiques of how penal institutions are increasingly governed through performance metrics, efficiency targets and hierarchical oversight (Bennett, 2016). It explores how these pressures shape the experiences of both prisoners and prison staff, creating a culture in which peer-led induction is more concerned with fulfilling managerial objectives than delivering substantive support. The findings suggest that prison staff, as well as prisoners, experience the constraining effects of managerialism caught between institutional mandates and the realities of working within a rigid, bureaucratic system. Ultimately, this chapter challenges the assumption that peer-led interventions function as positive and supportive tools, instead arguing that they reflect the shifting nature of penal power – where suffering is reorganised rather than alleviated. It highlights how power-sharing between prisoners and staff is not indicative of genuine empowerment but rather a mechanism through which control and disengagement is redistributed under the guise of responsibilisation.

Chapter 8 critically examines how the iatrogenic harms stemming from peer-led interventions are exacerbated by a fundamental absence of informed theoretical and evaluative grounding. It highlights how prison interventions, when implemented without a clear conceptual framework, risk failing to achieve their intended outcomes and may, in fact, cause harm. As Welsh and Rocque (2014, p. 262) assert, 'in the absence of sound theory, programmes stand little chance to bring about good and may even cause harm'. To consider this issue, the chapter introduces the concept of Programme Theory, which refers to the overarching theoretical model that explains how an intervention is expected to work (Funnell & Rogers, 2011). It explores how a lack of a clearly articulated Programme Theory – particularly in terms of evaluation and structured feedback mechanisms – has allowed peer-led induction to evolve without sufficient scrutiny.

The absence of systematic evaluation has not only obscured the deficiencies of these interventions but has actively contributed to their counterproductive effects rather than providing meaningful support to prisoners. The chapter argues that this persistence of ineffective interventions is a product of institutional path dependency where flawed schemes endure despite their failures. Furthermore, it advances penal institutions engaging in 'cargo cult science' (Feynman, 1974) by blindly replicating interventions based on assumed success rather than empirical evidence. This lack of oversight undermines the original supportive intentions of peer-led induction and gives rise to the array of unintended harms explored throughout this book. Finally, the chapter considers the necessity of developing a commensurate Programme Theory to inform future iterations of peer support interventions. It argues that penal policy fails to embed clear theoretical justifications for intervention models. This serves as an initial contribution towards reform, advocating for a shift away from intervention models that perpetuate harm and towards evidence-based approaches that genuinely support prisoner adaptation and well-being.

Chapter 9 reflects on the key findings of this book and its contribution to contemporary criminological inquiry, particularly within the context of the ongoing crisis in prisons. It situates the study within wider debates on penal governance, mental health and intervention effectiveness, offering a critical assessment of how peer-led induction has been positioned as a solution to systemic failures while, in reality, reinforcing institutional control and perpetuating unintended harms. The book has demonstrated how peer-led induction, rather than alleviating distress, frequently contributes to intervention iatrogenesis – the production of new harms or exacerbation of existing harms through intervention itself. This phenomenon underscores the ways in which prisoner support mechanisms can become mechanisms of coercion, responsibilisation and institutional disengagement rather than genuine support. The chapter also takes a philosophical and reflective approach, identifying the structural and procedural flaws that sustain ineffective interventions and examining how penal bureaucracy contributes to the endurance of failing programmes through path dependency and managerial inertia. Rather than evaluating programme efficacy, penal institutions often prioritise compliance with performance metrics, reinforcing the 'tick-box' culture that has allowed peer-led induction to persist despite its well-documented shortcomings. The book issues a direct challenge to penal policymakers, urging them to rethink intervention design in ways that prioritise prisoner well-being over institutional convenience.

To support this shift, the chapter calls for a departure from superficial, bureaucratically driven interventions towards evidence-based, needs-driven approaches that are rooted in rigorous Programme Theory and empirical evaluation. Future research must go beyond static assessments of intervention 'success' and instead adopt longitudinal and ethnographic methods to fully capture the lived experiences of prisoners navigating these programmes over time. At its core, this book has sought to underscore the reality that prisoners' lives matter and that, for peer interventions to serve their intended purpose, they must be built upon critical engagement, robust evaluation and a genuine commitment to prisoner well-being rather than bureaucratic expediency.

Chapter 2

'Pain Delivery': Enduring Issues and (Forgotten) Pains

> [Prisons provide] every imaginable means of infecting body and mind. (Bentham, cited in Bowring, 1843, pp. 351–352)

The mental health needs of those imprisoned in England and Wales have long been a critical consideration, especially regarding the impact of prison life on psychological well-being (Jewkes, 2007). While the state assumes responsibility for the mental health and safety of prisoners (HMCIP, 2017), the realities starkly contrast with government rhetoric, leading to the description of the prison system as being in a 'mental health crisis' (Allison, 2017). This crisis is often evidenced through self-harm and suicidal behaviours, especially during times of turmoil (Liebling, 1992; Lohner & Konrad, 2007).

This chapter examines the prevalence of mental health issues within the prison system, highlighting record levels of self-harm and suicidality. These issues, though unprecedented in scope, are rooted in long-standing problems exacerbated by failed reforms. Tracing the historical context, the chapter reviews key reports: Gladstone Committee (1895), the Prison System Enquiry (1922), the Woolf Report (1991) and the Bradley Report (2009), showing how policy failures and persistent issues have led to the current crisis in prison mental health. The chapter argues that, despite the decline of physical punishment, imprisonment still causes significant psychological distress (Crewe, 2011a, 2011b; Sykes, 1958), with prison continuing to serve as a mechanism for 'legitimated pain delivery' (Carlen, 1994, p. 136). While the penal system has evolved, pain remains intrinsic to imprisonment, especially during the initial stages such as reception into custody, where the experience of pain correlates strongly with adaptation and harm (Crewe et al., 2014; Liebling, 1995; Sapsford, 1983).The shift from overt coercive power to psychological power in contemporary prisons has resulted in new forms of suffering. This transition is explored through Foucault's concept of power and pain (Foucault, 1977) and its manifestation in modern penal systems, where psychological assessments and increased responsibilisation lead to iatrogenic suffering (Illich, 1975, 1976). The chapter further examines Sykes' (1958)

Navigating Mental Health in the Male Open Prison, 17–42

doi:10.1108/978-1-83549-706-720251002

framework of the core pains of imprisonment and Crewe's (2011a, 2011b) expansion of this framework to account for contemporary psychological distress, showing how the reconfiguration of penal power has compounded prisoner suffering, especially during the process of adaptation to prison life. Finally, the chapter explores the 'forgotten' pains associated with entry and adaptation to prison, particularly in open prisons. Foucault's concept of imprisonment as an attack on the psyche (Foucault, 1977) is examined, alongside Crewe's (2011a, 2011b) notion of 'tightness' in penal power, which shapes prisoner behaviour and exacerbates distress. Despite efforts to reform, the intrinsic pain of imprisonment persists, evolving in form but deepening the psychological suffering of prisoners.

Mental Health in Our Penal System

As of December 2024, the prison population sat at a figure of 85,373, with males accounting for 95% of this population. Between July and September 2024, there were 23,818 incidences of prisoner transfer, with 20,398 prisoners having at least one incidence of transfer. Both figures represent increases of 8% since the same period of 2023 (MOJ, 2025b). The overall statistics surrounding death in custody demonstrate that in the 12 months to September 2024, there were 317 deaths in prison custody, an increase of 4% from 304 deaths in the previous 12 months; of these deaths, 88 were self-inflicted (MOJ, 2025b). Looking at the long-term trend, the statistics are indicative of the mental health concerns and issues across England and Wales, with the total number of self-inflicted deaths in June 2009 standing at 63 and rising to the current figure. Considering the same period in relation to male self-inflicted death, there were a total of 61 self-inflicted deaths in 2009, rising by 36% to the figure of 83.

When considering the statistics surrounding self-harm in custody, they demonstrate a more harrowing picture, with a prisoner 'self-harming every ten minutes in jails across England and Wales' (Bulman, 2019). Overall, considering the male and female estate, there were a record high of 76, 535 incidences of self-harm in the 12 months to June 2024, a 19% increase from the previous 12 months, although one must caution that these are only the visible recorded incidents and there are likely to be many more that have remained undeclared, preventing the true extent of self-harm to be captured. There was a 13% increase in the rate of self-harm incidents per 1,000 prisoners in the 12 months to June 2024, with the rate now peaking at 876 incidents per 1,000 prisoners. However, there continue to be notable differences in self-harm trends by gender. There was an increase in the rate of self-harm incidents in male establishments to a new peak (up 20% to 664 incidents per 1,000 prisoners) and a decrease in the rate in female establishments (down 7% to 5,785 per 1,000 prisoners). The rate is more than eight times higher in female establishments than male establishments, down from more than 11 times higher in the previous 12 months. There was a decrease in the average number of incidents among those who self-harmed in female establishments, from 17.9 to 17.5, and a decrease in the rate of females self-harming (down 5% to 330 self-harming individuals per 1,000 prisoners). For males, there were increases in both the average number of incidents among those who self-harmed in male establishments (from 4.1 to 4.5) and the rate of individuals self-harming (up 11% to 149 self-harming individuals per 1,000 prisoners) with self-harm incidents requiring hospital attendance increasing in male establishments by 17% to 3,040 in the 12 months to June 2024 (MOJ, 2025b, 2025c). There is therefore a real need for focus on the male estate which this book adopts. Such a reality is, sadly, not a surprise. Rather, poor physical and mental health of prisoners has been an enduring and pervasive feature of the prison system over time. It has also been an ongoing concern of several investigations to which the chapter now turns.

The Gladstone Committee (1895)

The process of penal reform started with the Gladstone Report (1895) which Harding (1988, p. 592) argues 'the most considered statement of penal policy in this country' bringing about the 'inevitable end to a discredited system'. In the lead up to the committee's inception, an overarching argument was that the prison system in place was one that was symbolic of penal failure. The combination of this alongside increasing public and media sensitivity and pressure prompted the then Home Secretary, Herbert Asquith, to set up the committee to investigate and reform the prison system in England and Wales. This took place in the form of 35 committee sittings, spanning a total of 56 witnesses from a range of professions and agencies. The breadth of these testimonies provided a comprehensive understanding of the challenges facing the prison system.

The regime that prison administrator Edmund Du Cane had imparted to this point was founded on the notion that imprisonment was intended to deter offenders from further offences, which William Booth ascribed as ignoring 'the first essential of every system of punishment-reformation' (cited in Potter, 2019, p. xii). Du Cane represented the antithesis of a potential shift in penal philosophy to a reformatory position, which was more favourable in societal and political culture. He believed that reform should play a subsidiary role in the prison system. This 'stifled the institutional potential of the prison system' (Harding, 1988, p. 602).

The power of punitive public debate, the media and political cultures were a pivotal perpetuating factor in the shift in penal philosophy at the time the Gladstone Committee came to fruition. The Daily Chronicle in 1894 had delivered 'an articulate condemnation of the more severe physical and psychological features of the prison regime, [which] had touched the public's sensitivity to the issue' (Harding, 1988, p. 603). Of grave concern to the public, media, policymakers and prison staff was mental health it affirmed that 'among the prison population the ratio of insanity arising among persons sane on admission is not less than three times as great as that amongst the general population' (Cox & Marland, 2018, p. 707). The primary objections levied by critics centred on prison regime and operationalisation. Prisons at this point housed a large proportion of those who should have been in mental health institutions with adequate provisions to address such complex needs. The Chief Medical Officer of HMP Pentonville (in Gladstone, 1895) saw much value in the critics' viewpoint, observing the profoundly negative interaction of prison conditions and environment on prisoner mental health. The campaign against this regime drilled down on public populism, with their attitudes moving away from repressive deterrence and aspiring to something aligned with better prisoner outcomes, positive in nature. It condemned the often severe physical and psychological aspects of the prison regime (Potter, 2019). The media's role had been arguably integral in the shift in philosophy underpinning the reformatory position, as indeed the media's role to this very day is entangled with the climate of punishment.

Lushington (cited in Gladstone, 1895) perhaps best encapsulated the issues the committee had with the previous prison administration. He felt that their current approach was the antithesis of what the prison should do and how it should be run, noting that:

> I regard as unfavourable to reformation the status of a prisoner throughout his whole career; the crushing of self-respect, the starving of all moral instinct he may possess, the absence of all opportunity to do or receive a kindness. I believe that the true mode of reforming a man or restoring him to society is in exactly the opposite direction of all these. (cited in Gladstone, 1895, p. 8)

However, Lushington cautioned that aspiring to an operational and ideological vision departing from these institutional failures was an endeavour of folly, proclaiming '[t]his is a mere idea [...] It is quite impracticable in a prison. In fact, the unfavourable features that I have mentioned are inseparable from prison life' (Gladstone, 1895).

Theorists in ensuing years have proclaimed similar notions in that 'unpleasantness' and 'pain' are intrinsic to the concept of punishment and indeed the apparatus to mete it out (Bean, 1981; Goffman, 1961). The committee's investigations identified a range of issues within institutions of punishment, underpinning prison being painful for those imprisoned. Of particular concern was the lack of uniform treatment principles and institutional inconsistency (Gladstone, 1895, p. 6). The committee raised overcrowding in prisons, with the provision of accommodation not sufficient to house offenders. It questioned the rigidity of practices regarding visits and communications and the detrimental effects on prisoners of excessive and disproportionate punishments. There was criticism of unproductive labour as having no reformative value. They highlighted that isolation and confinement in work and association leads to moral and physical deterioration and the severe 'undesirable' deficiencies in the ability for prisoners to educate themselves. They also highlighted concerns over a lack of exercise and the grouping of all ages of male prisoners as undesirable and detrimental. In totality, these aspects contributed to the notions that '[p]rison life in itself is a potent cause in its [mental disorder/illness] development' (Gladstone, 1895, p. 33). All these identified issues were, and still are, associated with having a detrimental psychological effect upon those imprisoned. Warehousing of prisoners was significant, and people who should have been receiving care were instead subjected to criminalisation and control within a system devoid of any appropriate approach to the needs of those mentally ill. It is this warehousing that is arguably still evident in the current penal system when considering the levels of mental illness in prisons today.

The committee recognised substantial increases in instances of mental health disorder and illness among the offender population. Among the prison population, the ratio of insanity arising among persons apparently sane on admission was not less than three times as great as that among the general population of corresponding ages (Gladstone, 1895, pp. 48–49). Contributions from witnesses including prison staff, medical professionals and ex-prisoners further supported the position that imprisonment contributed to adverse mental health. There is perhaps no more severe manifestation of mental order and illness – and certainly no more final – than that of suicide. Gladstone (1895, p. 104) received profound observations that the number of suicides was out of proportion, acknowledging that the majority of suicides occur soon after an individual is received into custody and that 'the temptation to [commit suicide] becomes weaker the longer the time spent in prison'.

What was also of great concern, and still present in contemporary penology, is a lack of healthcare personnel to address the mental health concerns and issues of prisoners. Furthermore, the staff that were in place were beset by an absence of adequate experience in diagnosing and treating mental health disorders and requiring more personnel. This was especially important given that the volume of prisoner arrivals often made assessment of prisoners a 'hurried affair' (Gladstone, 1895, p. 177). Given the significant presence of mental disorder among the prison population, the deficiencies in medical support meant there was inadequate identification and treatment of them.

The many failings relating to the mental health of prisoners has led to concerns in the current system post Gladstone, regarding delivering safer custody in the prison estate. Safer custody is a term much vaulted, and broadly means the management of prisoners at risk of harm to self, to others and from others. Its roots can be traced back to the Prisons Act of 1877, referred to frequently by The Gladstone Committee. Of note is the way in which the term is applied to how prisons should operationalise the principles of safer custody and the antecedent from this time that resonates with today's sentiments is that:

> Regard shall be had to safe custody, but that every consideration shall be given to the treatment that is consistent with that safe custody and the discipline of the prison. (Gladstone, 1895, p. 366)

The commission was not deterred by the plethora of issues they identified nor daunted by negative perspectives surrounding tangible reform. They countered that while their description of prison life was negative, change for the better was possible. As a result, a much-remedied system was outlined in a series of recommendations to address the issues weighing down upon the penal systems. Their recommendations provided the foundations for the evolution of the prison system that we now recognise.

In addition to the specific issues relating to mental healthcare provision, the committee advanced further recommendations for increases in single-cell accommodations and a quicker admissions process. The committee proposed more discretion with visits and communications, greater interaction between support agencies and prisoners prior to release, the abolition of unproductive labour, the extension of association during work and leisure and productive industries to be developed, with a greater supply of books and better quality of education. The committee further proposed a more appropriate skill set in those staff engaging with prisoners. This was especially true concerning mental health, recommending all medical officers should have experience of special attention to mental disorder. The committee also called for confinement to be reduced and the level of punishments applied for refractory behaviours to be lessened alongside the first construction of what is recognised today as the Incentives and Earned Privileges (IEP) Scheme, when advancing that prisoners should be enabled to earn money throughout the course of their sentences.

These were all recommendations which were attempting to address a system that provided conditions 'absolutely opposed to mental, moral and physical health' (Potter, 2019, p. 337) of those housed within it and of the belief that modification could take place, transforming the prison into a system that is:

> . . .more elastic, more capable of being adapted to the special cases of individual prisoners, that discipline be, and treatment should be more effectually designed to maintain, stimulate or awaken the higher susceptibilities of prisoners. . ..and whenever possible to turn them out of prison better men and women, both physically and morally, than when they came in. (Gladstone, 1895, p. 8)

However, as the ensuing discussion demonstrates, this philosophy and the recommendations of Gladstone were sadly not realised and failed to provide appropriate improvements to regime, conditions and provision that are aligned with delivering positive outcomes for prisoner mental health and well-being.

The Prison System Enquiry Committee (1922)

Identifying progress in the prison system in the ensuing years post-Gladstone had proven to be difficult due to the secrecy that shrouded the penal estate (Gilligan & Pratt, 2003, p. 87). There had been no systematic enquiry since Gladstone despite plentiful opportunity to engage with the prison experiences of many men and women exposed to it. In response to this, the Executive of the Labour Research Department commissioned the Prison System Enquiry Committee. The object was not to table reform but discover fact through exploring the operation in the system as it stood and its results. It also represented an initial empirical recognition of transition between prisons interacting with the mental health of people who are imprisoned. A key benchmark to consider whether the recommendations of Gladstone had been implemented and their level of success, it was referred to as the 'the bible of prison reformers' by Margaret Fry of The Howard League (Harding, 1988).

Any optimism for a reformed and improved prison following the work of Gladstone was stifled by the findings of Hobhouse and Brockway (1922). The narrative of the enquiry became not one of progress and improvement but one of continued dissatisfaction and decline. Prison labour continued to lack choice, was unwaged, was devoid of training to support employment upon release and the work was degrading. Education provisions lacked competent teachers, there was little investment in education and education was restricted with a lack of materials and opportunity to go beyond the basics. Regarding communication, letters were delayed and censorship unnecessarily intrusive with visits infrequent and short in duration with the distances for family to travel excessive. The recommendations of the Gladstone committee had clearly not been realised (Hobhouse & Brockway, 1922). However, it was the evidence that 'denotes the bad effect of imprisonment upon health' (Hobhouse & Brockway, 1922, p. 253) that demonstrated the most concerning issues.

The findings identified initial reception to prison and adaptation as critical junctures in relation to the mental health of the population. This was illustrated by a large number of deaths following reception and the recognition that the experience of imprisonment and adaptation to it are intrinsically linked. They documented the greater tendency for suicide to be committed in the first week of imprisonment than at any subsequent period, that those under remand or awaiting sentence are more likely to commit suicide and that first-time prisoners display a greater liability to commit suicide.

The report highlighted the fact that good calibre medical staff are rarely attached or attracted to the prison service and that the staff that do exist are neither substantial enough in number to enable psychological study and treatment to be undertaken nor competent for such duties, with 'inadequacy' and 'amateurish' being terminologies applied to describe provision (Hobhouse & Brockway, 1922). In relation to insanity, the average rate occurring was nearly five times greater than that of the general population and increased from the time of the Gladstone Committee. Conclusions were also drawn in relation to suicide, finding that the features of the prison are the environmental influences of mental disorder, which also appear to cause suicide. The excessive nature of prison suicide was indicative of the prevalent nature of continued issues and decline:

> While [some] features of prison life may be held to be more particularly harmful, most of its defects reside in the more general principle on which the system as a whole is based. These defects appear to be the result of having set up as primary aims the ideas of retribution and deterrent punishment and of allowing. . .the working of the machine stands before any interest in the welfare of the imprisoned men and women. (Hobhouse & Brockway, 1922, p. 585)

This captures the acknowledgement of the tensions arising from the underlying philosophies of punishment. The rigours of prison life, the hopelessness, confinement, harsh attitude of staff, restrictions of prison and the shock of imprisonment were found to combine with the politicised institutional aims of the system to 'foster abnormal states of mind' (Hobhouse & Brockway, 1922, p. 534). A system of reform as conceived by Gladstone had evolved into one synonymous with regression rather than progression. This regression further continued, culminating in a series of prison disturbances across the prison estate in England and Wales, which visibly expressed the distress of those imprisoned.

The Woolf Report (1991)

Following the prison enquiry, the next key report that focused on the enduring conditions of imprisonment came in response to a wave of serious prison riots across the penal estate in England and Wales in the form of the Woolf Report (1991). As an admirable and landmark investigation, the Woolf Report confirmed the continuing decline in prison conditions and healthcare provision across the penal estate and proposed a plethora of recommendations for change. These included the need for improved healthcare provision and the need for equivalence of physical and mental healthcare with the general population. It was labelled as the most important report since the Gladstone Report of 1895. Yet, the Woolf Report signified that optimism stemming from Gladstone proved to be unfounded regarding remedying the issues in the prison system. It highlighted an absence of substantive progress alongside a continued demise of the rehabilitative ideal and ethos, which left the prison system rudderless with no clear purpose, despite previous efforts to provide one. In this latter part of the 20th century, the prison system had become a model of containment, papering over the cracks of the conditions of imprisonment. This existed alongside the age-old operational strain brought about by incessant growth of the penal population, the physical degradation of prisons themselves and the primary risk-averse focus of the administration which operated with blinkers on, seeing only security and dangerousness of prisoners (Player & Jenkins, 1994).

Prisons across England and Wales were beset by these issues, and there was a sense of malaise in them until a series of prison riots played out across the penal estate. The most visible of these riots was at HMP Strangeways in 1990. Serious riots broke out further afield across another five prisons, reporting 30 more institutions experiencing some form of disturbance across England and Wales (Player & Jenkins, 1994). These riots, and riots that have occurred throughout the history of the penal system, are not what can be classed as isolated, one-off events. However, although not a new phenomenon, the way in which riots are constructed, defined and responded to has evolved over time. They are manifestations of the multitude of failings and issues that teem through the penal system and only cease once appropriately addressed. The prisoners in these riots sought to have their voices heard to mobilise collectively to achieve what Sykes (1958, p. 110) would describe as a 'logical step in a pattern of repeated social change'. These disturbances provided explicit and graphic imagery and evidence of the issues in the prison system, which reached the living rooms of people across the country, leaving an imprint of disorder, discontent, loss of control and disarray.

Woolf and Tumin (1991) recognised that justice was not aligned with the notion of treating prisoners with humanity. His definition of justice moved beyond the confines of previous investigations as well as bureaucratic procedure and due process to encompass the conditions inside the prison, spelling out that 'if the prison service contains that prisoner in conditions which are inhumane or degrading then a punishment of imprisonment which was justly imposed will result in injustice' (Woolf & Tumin, 1991, p. 10.19). This in turn led to the documented outpourings to facilitate change as outlined. These resonated with the notions of Sykes (1958) who had earlier written about differing pains associated with the experience of imprisonment for those imprisoned and ways in which they manifest. Woolf was able to go beyond the facile notions proffered by prison officials positioning life sentenced prisoners with nothing to lose and those with psychological issues being 'carceral riot-bombs' who went off, as the embodiment of the unrest.

What Woolf and Tumin (1991) uncovered were a range of systemic causes that were to the detriment of both the prisons and the prisoners, in terms of their mental health. Yet more disturbingly, this provided further illustration of a system that was continuing to exhibit the same issues that had harmed it over time. These issues had continued to worsen despite reformatory practices in the years post-Gladstone. Prisoner perspectives highlighted the overcrowded physical conditions, the unconstructive nature of the regime, the lack of respect with which they were treated, the destructive effects of imprisonment and the institution on their family ties and visitation. The lack of staff, lack of staff training, hierarchical divides and lack of direction and leadership were also identified. The endemic nature of these issues is encapsulated in the build-up of this tension being 'like pressure in a pressure cooker'. Woolf also recognised immediately that it was 'clear that there will remain for the foreseeable future a significant problem for the prison service in accommodating mentally disordered offenders' (Woolf & Tumin, 1991, p. 257). He also called for equivalence of care and research into the effectiveness of the mental health provisions already in place, which were significantly under-evaluated.

Overall, Woolf called for a shift in the philosophy of punishment and purpose of imprisonment, proposing a rehabilitative approach moving forward. This involved departing from the reformative model whereby offenders were sent to prison for treatment and moving towards a form of individualised and responsibilised self-help, whereby tools such as educational, vocational and therapeutic opportunities would be provided to the prisoner to address their offending behaviour, mental health and well-being issues and to prepare them for release and. However, the gravitas attached to the report was a superficial appraisal despite the furore catalysing a renewed vigour to steer the rudderless prison ship towards a clear vision. This was predicated on riding the wave of a more 'radical justice approach' under a more liberal Home Secretary in the form of Kenneth Clarke though to expect him to shake himself free from the shackles of what came before would be a tough proposition. Moreover, society had heard it all before. Despite the circumstances that brought about the review, one would have been forgiven for expecting it to show improvements across the board given the findings and recommendations of previous reports and the significant period elapsing since. This historical review, however, demonstrated that almost 100 years after the Gladstone Committee carried out its investigation, Woolf and Tumin's had evidenced the same issues of Gladstone (1985) and Hobhouse and Brockway (1922). It was clear to see that the extent, prevalence and enduring nature of the issues in the prison system had continued. This raised the question as to what would be different this time? The answer was nothing, but this was not for want of trying.

This time, the opportunity to implement Woolf's Gladstone-esque proposals, was stifled when the media, public and political realms collided once again but in stark contrast to the outcomes of this interaction 100 years earlier. Crime received limited attention as a political issue before 1970 and there being a general cross-party liberal consensus, which included proposals to reduce the use of imprisonment citing concerns of effectiveness to rehabilitate prisoners and their operational cost. However, this gradually started to fracture, leading up to the 1979 election with the roots of a forthcoming punitive turn firmly in place (Pratt et al., 2005). Crime was highlighted as an issue causing a current of social anxiety among the public, which in turn presented a vote-securing opportunity for government, seeking to alleviate this fear through a shift away from liberal principles to the implementation of a punitive ethos and justice policy.

For radical justice reforms post-Woolf, the window of opportunity proved to be short lived as Clarke was succeeded by Michael Howard in 1993. Presenting as someone embracing a populist law and order stance, he crushed any vigour with an approach that put 'prisons as the solution to crime [...] they should hold greater numbers not fewer, conditions of detention should be more austere not less' (House of Commons, 1993). Containment, punishment and deterrence were all back on the scene with no mention of rehabilitation or fairness and completely eradicated any hope of an improved prison system in England and Wales.

The Bradley Report (2009)

Alongside this evaporation of hope, the late 20th and early 21st century yielded a wealth of research demonstrating that prisoners continue to suffer from poor mental health (De Vigianni, 2006). It signified endangered mental health, evidencing that anxiety, depression and the stress of prison, the prison environment and its rules and daily regimes affect many prisoners (Bradley, 2009; Crewe & Liebling, 2017; Graham, 2007; Jewkes, 2007; WHO, 1998). The next significant report off the government production line was The Bradley Report (2009), which examined the treatment of individuals with mental health problems and learning disabilities in the criminal justice system, emphasising the pressing need for reform. While its overarching goal was to explore alternatives to custody for offenders with mental health issues, it also highlighted the significant ways in which imprisonment exacerbates psychological distress. Bradley built upon the foundations laid by the Woolf Report (1991) and other preceding inquiries, advocating for a fundamental shift in how prisons handle mental health. A core focus was on achieving equivalence between prison healthcare and that available in the community, recognising that failure to meet this standard constituted a violation of prisoners' basic rights (Exworthy et al., 2012).

At the time of the Bradley Report, the prevalence of mental illness in prisons was stark. Over 90% of prisoners were estimated to have at least one psychiatric disorder, such as psychosis, neurosis, personality disorder or substance dependency, with rates dramatically exceeding those found in the general population (Singleton et al., 1998, 2001). The report underscored the dire need for improved screening, early intervention and continuity of care, recognising that many individuals with mental health conditions entered custody without proper diagnosis or treatment. Despite the government's commitment to addressing these disparities, progress remained slow, and the reality of prison life continued to undermine efforts to support prisoner well-being (Durcan et al., 2014).

The Bradley Report detailed the historical failures of prison mental healthcare, situating them within a broader pattern of neglect and systemic dysfunction. While the Reed Review (1992) had previously called for a more integrated, multi-agency approach to managing mentally disordered offenders, implementation remained inconsistent, leading to significant gaps in service provision. The lack of trained medical personnel within prisons was a longstanding issue, with healthcare staffing levels remaining inadequate and training often insufficient to address the complexity of prisoner mental health needs. In-reach mental health services, which were designed to provide specialist support within prisons, faced overwhelming demand, with referral rates increasing exponentially (Exworthy et al., 2012). These pressures meant that services intended for the most acutely unwell were often diverted, leaving many prisoners without appropriate care. The report also identified deficiencies in mental health screening processes, noting that many prisoners with serious psychological conditions were not properly assessed upon entry into custody. The reliance on non-mental health-trained prison staff to identify at-risk individuals further exacerbated the problem, as many officers lacked the expertise to recognise or respond effectively to signs of distress. Although training programmes had been introduced, their effectiveness was limited by poor attendance and operational constraints, preventing officers from participating (Bradley, 2009). The result was a system where early warning signs were frequently missed, leading to preventable crises, including self-harm and suicide (HMCIP, 2007).

Despite recognising some positive developments in mental health, Bradley remained sceptical about their overall impact, arguing that meaningful change had yet to materialise. The government had introduced initiatives aimed at improving mental health in custody, such as the Offender Health Strategy and the Improving Health, Supporting Justice framework, yet these often lacked adequate funding and strategic oversight (Durcan et al., 2014). The principle of equivalence between prison and community healthcare, which had been a central policy aim since 1990, was far from being realised. Prisoners consistently faced barriers to accessing appropriate healthcare (Bradley, 2009).

One of the most pressing concerns raised in the report was the failure of existing policies to prevent the deterioration of mental health among prisoners. The prison environment was identified as a key factor in exacerbating psychological distress. The impact was reflected in alarmingly high rates of self-harm and suicidality, which had been on an upward trajectory (Walton et al., 2025). Although efforts had been made to improve suicide prevention and safer custody measures, these initiatives were increasingly undermined by austerity-driven budget cuts and a broader shift towards punitive penal policies. As Ismail (2020, 2022) recognises, prisons are places of punishment, yet the austerity measures transcend merely the loss of liberty, compounding mental health issues and thus extending punishment. The violence of austerity had not only deepened inequalities within the prison system but also severely limited the capacity to provide effective mental healthcare (Bulman, 2019).

The Bradley Report acknowledged that mental health was moving up the policy agenda, with increased governmental recognition of the need for reform. However, it cautioned against assuming that rhetorical commitments would translate into tangible improvements. Historically, mental health policy in prisons had often been reactive rather than proactive, with new strategies emerging in response to crises rather than as part of a sustained commitment to change. This pattern of policy by press release reflected the wider tendency for governments to prioritise public and political sentiment over evidence-based reform (Bradley, 2009). While the Bradley Report sought to challenge this cycle, its findings suggested that significant obstacles remained in the path towards meaningful progress.

There was a need for financial investment and also a cultural shift in how the criminal justice system approached mental illness. Without such a shift, prisons would continue to act as default holding facilities for those with complex mental health needs, perpetuating cycles of distress. Ultimately, the Bradley Report reinforced a troubling reality: despite decades of research and policy recommendations, prisoners with mental health conditions remained among the most neglected populations in the criminal justice system. The promise of equivalence in healthcare had yet to be fulfiled, and the structural deficiencies in prison mental health provision continued to place thousands of individuals at risk (Exworthy et al., 2012). Without sustained political will and substantial investment, the issues highlighted in Bradley's work were destined to persist, ensuring that prisons remained sites of psychological suffering. The cycle of neglect and inadequate reform, which had been a defining feature of prison mental health policy for over a century, showed no signs of abating. Mental health has long been ascribed aims, purpose and direction in the penal estate through a raft of policy initiatives yet fails to deliver the results it promises to yield, namely the improved mental health of the prison population.

Despite the Bradley Report's call for improved mental health provisions in prisons, as did all the reports discussed, the reality remains that imprisonment is often the cause or exacerbator of psychological distress. While policymakers continue to frame mental healthcare as a reform issue, they fail to address a deeper truth: prisons are not just sites of treatment failure, but active producers of suffering. Beyond the lack of adequate mental health services, the very structure of incarceration operates as a system of control that inflicts psychological pain on those within it. As Carlen (1994, p. 136) argues, the prison remains a 'mechanism for legitimated pain delivery', where suffering is not incidental but inherent to the institution. This creates the impression of government making 'policy by press release' (Bulman, 2019; Stevens et al., 2025) and as such our prisons find themselves in the position that they are in today in the midst of a mental health crisis. To fully grasp the persistent mental health crisis in prisons, it is necessary to examine how power functions within these institutions, shaping prisoners' experiences and reinforcing systems of control. The next section explores how the shift from overt coercion to psychological governance has deepened the pains of imprisonment rather than alleviating them.

Prisons, Power and Pain

> [. . .] in examining the pains of imprisonment as they exist today, it is imperative that we go beyond the fact that severe bodily suffering has long since disappeared as a significant aspect of the custodian's regime, leaving behind a residue of apparently less acute hurts such as the loss of liberty, the deprivation of goods and services, the frustration of sexual desire and so on. These deprivations or frustrations of the modern prison may be the acceptable or unavoidable implications of imprisonment, but we must recognise that they can be just as painful as the physical maltreatment which they have replaced. Such attacks on the psychological level are less easily seen than a sadistic beating, a pair of shackles on the floor, or the caged man on a treadmill, but the destruction of the psyche is no less fearful than bodily affliction. (Sykes, 1958, p. 64)

As punishment evolved in society, there was a shift from punishment that inflicted physical harm to one that punished the soul and the psychological well-being of those convicted, and to this, the concept of power remains central (Shammas, 2017). While contemporary society has largely seen the replacement of physical and overt forms of punishment, through the softening of penal power, the effects of imprisonment continue to impose a range of pains and suffering, culminating in psychological distress (Crewe, 2011a, 2011b; Sykes, 1958). Despite the aforementioned efforts to improve the penal system over time, prison is synonymous with pain delivery. Significantly, there are certain stages of a sentence of imprisonment where this pain of imprisonment is experienced more profoundly, such as reception into custody. Pain at this juncture has a considerable effect upon adaptation to prison life (Crewe et al., 2014; Liebling, 1999; Sapsford, 1983) with Liebling (1995, p. 183) asserting that research shows a 'clear link between the pain of imprisonment and harm'.

Power

According to Matthews (2014, p. 43), 'every facet of law and order is infused with power…from the interpersonal to the structural, power operates at every level'. Power here is as defined by Wrong (2017, p. 2) to be 'the capacity of some persons to produce intended and foreseen effects on others'. Prison is an institution which typifies and illustrates the complex entanglement of power relations embedded within its walls. Foucauldian theory (1975, 1977) is founded on interest in the different ways that power manifests itself and its impact upon attitudes and actions. It conceptualises power as embodied within the creation and operation of the modern prison and those within it (Matthews, 2014). Elias (1984, p. 251) states:

> In fact, what we call power is an aspect of a relationship, of every human relationship. It has something to do with the fact that people as groups or as individuals can withhold or monopolize what others need- food, love, meaning, protection from attack (security) as well as knowledge and some other things.

In this sense, prison is therefore the monopolisation of what others need, which feeds into the deprivation thesis offered by Sykes (1958), all of which combine to contribute to diminish well-being of those who are imprisoned. In keeping with the traditions of many penal scholars' discussion of prison and power would be incomplete without an acknowledgement of Foucault. While this is appropriate in this case, the work of Elias is just as relevant and important, and, rather than existing separately to one another, their theorisation can be reconciled to evidence hybrid theory of re-configured penal power and punishment. The first convergence between Foucault and Elias is that they both agree with the proposition that power is everywhere, and both postulate the omnipresence of the phenomena of power (Spierenburg, 2004).

The prison system in England and Wales evidences two distinct constructions of power: 'hard and soft'. As aforementioned, just as punishment has evolved in its construction and enactment, so too has its primary mechanism, the prison. Crewe (2009, 2011b) argues there is hard power, synonymous with historic prison practices and often aligned with coercion and conditions of brutality, degradation and austerity with attempts to create an overt culture of fear, to be punitive and dehumanising. The shift from these practices – just like those in punishment more generally since the 18th century which Foucault (1977) claimed – was illustrative of incarceration as a punishment of the soul and no longer primarily the body can also be said to be indicative of forming what Elias would term a civilising process. Here, Elias' carving of the meat illustration can be invoked as an analogy. There used to be the spectacle of carving the meat in front of guests at the dinner table, but over time, this spectacle was rendered as a distasteful insult to civilised sensibility. The carving doesn't stop however, as people still eat meat. Rather, distasteful is removed to behind the scenes of social life. This can be applied to power and pain. There is no longer the meting out of hard power in overt, physical and brutal, degrading pain in front of the eyes of the public and prison population. This is now unpalatable. However, pain is still inflicted. Power is instead veiled with pain being administered covertly and in psychological forms. So here the theorisations of Foucault, that power has changed in its form, resonates with Elias' theorisation (Elias, 1978).

While prisons have moved from their historic position of hard power, in the contemporary system different security category prisons evidence differing applications of power. The prison system today has been characterised by a reconfigured penal power to one based on 'soft power' and the open prison of today is without doubt the most extreme and illustrative example of such a power application. This soft power is actioned through a range of policies and procedures that emphasise the prisoner self-regulating their behaviour and taking on the responsibility of doing so, alongside the responsibility to drive the addressing of their offending behaviour, being pro-social members of the prison environment and community, and being accountable for their failings in achieving these elements. As Alford (2000, pp. 141–142) argues, 'we should not, however, confuse the decentralization of power with the transformation of power'. The decentralised power applied is not necessarily more subtle, just much less visible. Arguably as Foucault (1977, p. 308) states, 'the most important effect, perhaps of the carceral system [...] is that it makes the power to punish appear natural and legitimate, at least to lower the threshold of tolerance for penalty'. Inter alia, the monolithic structure of power constantly punishes, and everyone thinks it is normal.

Sykes' Pains of Imprisonment (1958)

> Lying somewhere between the total annihilation of the offender on one hand and warning or forgiveness on the other, imprisonment is generally viewed as the appropriate consequence of most serious crimes. (Sykes, 1958, p. 9)

It is in this sense the prison is symbolic of the application of state power to punish and exclude. Prior to this assertion by Sykes, there had been a number of historical commentators that had identified the negative impact of imprisonment. Dickens (1842/1883, pp. 678–679) lamented the imprisonment as 'cruel and wrong' and recognised anxiety and despair among prisoners while Mayhew (1862, p. 127) identified 'intense misery' from being 'hemmed in by four white walls'. Such characterisations of the profound detrimental impact upon the mental health and well-being of those imprisoned are further reflected in the aforementioned consideration of the reports into the prison.

Sykes (1958) recognised the value in understanding prison life. This was especially important during an era of supposed enlightenment, when changes to the aims of imprisonment and its operation were introduced with a limited understanding of their outcome for prisoners. This presence of a lack of understanding in the face of change is something that has endured. Sykes, however, was able to offer a framework that illustrated how the prison institution applied their power towards the prisoner and define the experience of imprisonment and its impact on the prisoner. He did so through five deprivations that he argued characterised prison life referred to as 'The Pains of Imprisonment'. In doing so, Sykes (1958, p. 64) acknowledged that the 'deprivations or frustrations of the modern prison may indeed be the acceptable or unavoidable implications of imprisonment, but we must recognize the fact that they can be just as painful as the physical maltreatment which they have replaced'. These deprivations and frustrations in the prison environment threaten the prisoners' sense of self and self-efficacy. The issues surrounding incarceration, including those described thus far, consistently exhibited across the penal estate and distinctive to the penal environment, were the combining factors that determined prison culture and how it is experienced. For Sykes and subsequently Goffman (1961), the prison was a system that was a largely autonomous monolith, cut off from the outside wider society. Goffman (1961) viewed the prison as a total institution where a cohort of people, sharing same characteristics and cut off from society, lived together in an enclosed and prescribed way of life.

The primary deprivation on the prisoner that Sykes described was the *removal and restriction of liberty*. Coyle (1994, p. 27) indicates the profoundly negative impact of this deprivation when he notes that 'losing one's liberty is one of the most traumatic experiences an individual is likely to ever undergo'. However, this restriction of liberty is not just the incapacitation of a person by placing them in prison. There is a raft of further measures within the prison that re-enforce the loss of liberty, such as cellular accommodation and military style movements around the prison. The deprivation of liberty erodes the ties binding family and friends, challenging the support network of those imprisoned. Although many prisons have procedures and policies in place for such routine aspects of day-to-day life to facilitate them, they remain restrictive, diluting their benefits. Calls and mails are monitored and visits dehumanising. This deprivation is often experienced most acutely by those in custody for the first time and can be extended to those transitioning between prisons (HMIP, 2015).

The second deprivation is the *deprivation of goods and services*. Sykes (1958) observed that prisoners will inevitably experience material deprivation and restriction, whether that be tobacco, alcohol, a varied diet alongside individualised clothing, furnishings and privacy. Societal cultures, especially in the contemporary Western world, place a great degree of importance on material goods, and they have a strong interaction with a person's identity. And they also serve as a symbol of status and their deprivation serves to diminish the sense of self. As such, the revocation of ability to acquire or enjoy such goods and services is a profound loss, symbolic of a corrosive attack upon the individual's personality and psyche.

Sykes provided a third deprivation, being that of *heterosexual relationships*. While the principle of deprivation is valid, Sykes did not recognise the deprivation as one that could be ascribed to homosexual prisoners, and he argued that the deprivation of heterosexual relations created 'latent homosexual tendencies'

(Shammas, 2017). However, there is the notion that enforced celibacy could cause psychological distress; therefore, this pain is expanded to include all sexual relationships across sexual orientations. Enforced celibacy experienced during imprisonment, according to Sykes, was a source of tension and anxiety and also clouded the individual's sense of self image and identity.

Sykes fourth pain is the *deprivation of autonomy*, which can also include a restriction to the level of control that a prisoner can exert over a situation to which they are subjected. The rules and regulations that prisoners are subjected to erode the most basic decisions that one makes about when and what to eat, when they can move and to where, and even extends to controlling their bodily functions (Sykes, 1958). For Sykes, the harm stemming from a lack of autonomy enacted through forced acts of deference reduced prisoners to what Shammas (2017) later recognised as a 'childlike state', again interacting with diminished identity. In this sense, the prisoner becomes a passive being upon whom things are inflicted; prison is 'done to' them. The provision of increased prisoner autonomy in the contemporary prison system does not necessarily mitigate this pain and continues to be cited as a source of psychological distress among prisoners.

The final and potentially most impacting pain for those entering and transitioning into prison settings is the *deprivation of security*. The prison system is one portrayed in media and discourse as synonymous with violence, bullying, threatening behaviour and sexual assault, often against a backdrop of substance use and dependence, which underpins insecurity. In the prison system of England and Wales, there are consistently reported highs in violent acts within prison with prisoners in close quarters, whether sharing cells or in other prison activities, with those with complex needs and with histories of violent and aggressive behaviours (Shammas, 2017). As Sykes argues, such conditions are a prominent source of anxiety and distress among prisoners, promoting fear and ontological insecurity attacking the prisoner's sense of self and identity. Goffman (1961) built upon Sykes' pains, by demonstrating how the institution removed the prisoner from life as they knew it and the outside world. This process of deconstructing the prisoner's identity involved the issuing of numbers as identification, prison uniforms, removal of contact with the outside world and the altering of physical appearance. Sykes argued that the pain of imprisonment, although obviously profound, can however be substantially reduced by social interaction, a notion particularly key when considering the role of peer support in supporting prisoner adaptation to prison.

While Sykes' (1958) work remains prominent as the founding conceptualisation of the issues underpinning distress in prisoners, the penal landscape is one that is ever evolving. As such, Sykes' framework is also one that, by default, requires adaptation and expansion. Earlier in this chapter, there was an emphasis on the changing nature of the penal system over time. It also stressed that such change should not necessarily be associated with success. That said, the contemporary prison estate in England and Wales is one that has nonetheless changed with this reconfiguration. As Toch (1977, cited in Johnson & Toch, 1982, p. 18) states, despite the vast extent of the pains that Sykes describes:

> ...it has become increasingly obvious that the pains of imprisonment are not uniform or constant. Different personal needs shared by prisoners, in turn produce different perceptions of prison environments and different reactions to imprisonment. One man's (or woman's) meat can indeed be another's poison; Prisons possess diverse ecologies and house diverse populations; transactions of prisoners make for a complex mosaic of stress and adaptation.

Emanating from the changes in the penal system are changes in the extent to which the pains identified by Sykes are experienced but also to a range of contemporary pains which go beyond the confines of Sykes' foundation.

Revisiting the Pains of Imprisonment: A Contemporary Insight

As established, the infliction of pain is no longer an explicit aim of punishment. Indeed, reform and enlightenment have seen efforts to improve the experience of imprisonment. However, pain is very much omnipresent across the prison estate, and it is this pain and frustration that has emerged iatrogenically, as an unintended consequence from the institutional policies and techniques of contemporary penal power (Bowling, 2011). It exists alongside their historic counterparts, albeit different in origin, impact and feel. This is illustrated when considering the typology of the total institution advanced by Goffman (1961) and in place during Sykes' theorisation. It is not one that can be wholly applied to the open prison estate, where individuals are no longer cut off from wider society or in a fully formal administered way of life, by virtue of both working and having home releases into the community among a culture of self-governance within the prison.

Crewe (2011a) identifies three categories of the contemporary pains of imprisonment that have arisen from the ashes of historic applications of hard power and the transition to perceived soft power: (i) the pains of uncertainty and indeterminacy; (ii) psychological assessment and (iii) self-government. All are mutually re-enforcing, entangled and experienced acutely in the open prison estate.

The Pains of Uncertainty and Indeterminacy

While Crewe considers uncertainty and indeterminacy together, given the deleterious and often more profound impact of what he describes as the tyrannical nature of the indeterminate sentence upon the experience of imprisonment, this chapter delineates them and considers uncertainty as a concept situated across sentence types and lengths. Indeed, many of the ideas presented are transferable across these elements.

All prisoners, regardless of sentence, experience anxiety about their future while navigating a present governed by shifting penal power. This is particularly evident in open prisons, where prisoners are given more autonomy but remain under constant scrutiny. Crewe argues that modern imprisonment blends 'soft' and 'hard' power – offering greater responsibility to prisoners while maintaining coercive control. In an open prison context, this dynamic creates confusion, as staff are either unable or unwilling to provide clear guidance, leaving prisoners in what Crewe (2011a, p. 515) describes as a 'fog of uncertainty'. The knowledge that harsher measures can be imposed at any time adds to their insecurity, fostering ontological insecurity and poor mental health outcomes (Crewe, 2011a; Giddens, 1984).

Open prison prisoners often feel they are 'treading on eggshells', fearing that minor infractions – real or perceived – could undo years of progress and result in a sudden return to closed conditions. Some believe they are set up to fail, as institutions weigh small mistakes more heavily than sustained good behaviour. This unpredictability is worsened by inconsistencies in how rules and regulations are applied. The softening of penal power, rather than fostering stability, has led to greater unpredictability, leaving prisoners uncertain about their status and interactions with staff.

The Pains of Psychological Assessment

Psychology has become central to modern prisons, particularly in open institutions, where risk assessment dictates key decisions on temporary release, recategorisation and rehabilitation programmes. As such, prison psychology has morphed from an offering to alleviate psychological distress among the prison population to 'a primary role as the providers of expert risk assessment' (Maruna, 2011b, p. 672). The processes of such psychological assessment in a penal world dominated by risk management are omnipresent in the lived experience of the prisoner and act as a powerful tool in determining their future, with the wielding of this psychological power often creating psychological distress to prisoners. It is often said that the pen is mightier than the sword, and this is apparent in the experience of prisoners who regularly express the perception that psychological reports, while often framed as supporting rehabilitation, are impersonal and intrusive, designed more for risk management than genuine self-exploration (Maruna, 2011b). Prisoners feel that reports misrepresent them, removing context, compassion and nuance. In the open prison estate, this scrutiny is heightened, as prisoners seeking release must demonstrate 'progress' in ways that align with institutional expectations rather than their authentic self-development.

Rather than alleviating distress, psychological assessments have become a tool of control, compelling prisoners to conform to prescribed behavioural expectations. Many feel pressured to adopt a 'shadow self' to meet assessment criteria, distorting their identity. Open prison prisoners are acutely aware that psychological reports can influence their future, with subjective assessments carrying long-term consequences. While not overtly coercive, this psychological oversight exerts significant power, adding to prisoners' anxiety and self-doubt as they attempt to navigate a system that demands compliance yet remains ambiguous and inconsistent in its judgements.

The Pains of Self-Government

Prisons have shifted from overt control to a Foucauldian model of self-regulation, particularly in open institutions, where prisoners are expected to exercise autonomy and responsibility for their rehabilitation (Rose, 2000). In open prisons, this shift is stark – prisoners move from a regimented environment to one where they must manage their own progress, often with minimal staff support. A further concern is that some prisoners do not have the skills to adapt to this level of autonomy or take time to adapt, which is understandable given that prisoners most likely will have spent prolonged periods in higher security closed prisons, where regime and control are more prescribed and directed. This transition creates anxiety, as prisoners must navigate ambiguous expectations while knowing that any misstep, no matter how minor, could lead to their removal back to closed conditions. Placing such men into conditions where what is appropriate is more loosely defined creates tense and fearful prisoners tiptoeing through their day-to-day life, cowering from the looming threat of a punishment.

There becomes a paradox: prisoners are no longer merely subjects of discipline but agents of their own incarceration. Some resent this shift, while others struggle with the skills needed to adapt. The blurred boundaries between staff authority and prisoner autonomy create a precarious state where prisoners live in fear of failing to meet unstated or inconsistent expectations. In open prisons, where personal responsibility is emphasised, this fear is particularly acute – rather than fearing just staff, prisoners fear their own potential missteps. This makes imprisonment even more psychologically demanding, as prisoners must constantly engage in the performativity of responsibility while grappling with the uncertainties of their own progress.

Forgotten (Transition Specific) Pains

Context is important, and a further range of pains have been identified that go beyond both Sykes' and Crewe's theorisations. Such pains can be applied to differing types and contexts of 'custody' and 'imprisonment'. Shammas (2014) has previously sought to consider the proliferation of pain further in the context of the open prison, terming them the 'pains of freedom'. While his conceptualisations around confusion, anxiety and boundlessness, ambiguity and responsibilisation have some degree of transferability to the conceptualisations this book advances – they are very much anchored to the context of freedom and the tensions navigating the tightrope between the establishment and freedom related activity. This chapter now considers a further five additional pains of imprisonment; *entry shock*, *fear of the unknown*, *lack of social support*, *physical environment* and *fear and nervousness about release* (Jones, 2007), which are directly experienced by those in the open estate in the context of transferring, transitioning and adapting to the establishment.

Entry shock is described as 'the turmoil individuals face during their initial period of incarceration when they enter the criminal justice system' (Jones, 2007, p. 22). This notion is often applied to those making their initial entry to custody from their status of liberty. The shock element is due to the suddenness of this transition and often manifests through the high levels of self-harm and suicide that prisoners experience in the early stage of admission (Blaauw et al., 1998; Ingram et al., 1997). However, it is argued that this is also experienced for those transferring between institutions. Prisoners go through a reception process when entering prison which signifies the start of a number of 'abasements, degradations, humiliations and profanations', a process that is the source of acute psychological stress for the prisoner (Goffman, 1961, p. 23). Although this may be experienced more acutely upon initial entry into custody, the prisoner will have to go through this process of mortification as they progress through the system on arrival at every prison they arrive at with the revisitation of this process reactivating this stress. This is due to it disrupting the prisoner's adaptation to the penal world and returning them to a position of liminality whereby they are overwhelmed by the introduction of a new regime and new surroundings detached from their comfort zone (Caird, 1974).

Jewkes and Laws (2020, p. 4) assert that it takes 'time to become accustomed to, and a common narrative [...] that confinement could be emotionally turbulent, especially during the early stages, when a liminal "state of being" meant the subject moving through a period of instability or chaos, to one of tolerance or even transformation and reinvention'. Liminality has enduring legacies in the anthropological conceptualisations. As a sociologically valuable notion, 'liminality' refers to the middle stage of any ritual process that can be decanted into three analytically distinct stages and during which a person transitions from one social position to another (Van Gennep, 1960; Turner, 1967). Wels et al. (2011) surmise that during the middle phase of this process, the individuals involved are described being 'no longer' and simultaneously also 'not yet'. It is thus an ambiguous phase; liminal personae are 'neither here nor there; they are betwixt and between the positions assigned and arrayed by law, custom, convention, and ceremonial' (Turner, 1967, p. 95).

This can be associated with a differing pain, the *fear of the unknown* (Jones, 2007). Again, this is experienced most acutely during the initial stages of any element of the criminal justice system when levels of uncertainty are at their peak. In its simplest form, it is often caused by a distinct lack of information and awareness about the individual's situations and surroundings, and it is especially evident when transferring and adapting to a new institution, regime and conditions. Here, the apprehensive prisoner becomes overwhelmed, and the uncertainty continues when going beyond the institution and factoring in the prisoner concerns about family, friends and support. All these serve to increase stress among the prisoner, and this fear will accompany them throughout custody, especially when considering the idea that prisoners are objects to whom prison is done with little to no agency in the decision-making processes that shape how custody is experienced.

A further pain of relevance is a *loss of social support* (Jones, 2007). This is not to be considered in the context of detachment from the outside world due to institutional demands and barriers. Rather, this is considered in the context of the open prison whereby those prisoners transferring to the new prison are removed from the support networks and relationships that they have developed over time with other prisoners. Just as relationships with the outside world are severed with separation from family and communication limited, the same then occurs in the penal world among peers when they transfer. Loss of support in this sense is linked to suicidal behaviour and self-harm (Liebling, 1999) and can have devastating effects on the ability of the prisoner to navigate the new penal environment.

An often-overlooked pain is the experience of the *physical environment* (Jones, 2007), not only of the prison itself but also an appreciation of how the prisoner is transported to their new establishment. Of course, there are the enduring austere and squalid conditions that prisoners live in throughout the estate, yet the exposure to these in open prison is much more limited due to the amount of time out of cell and away from the physical confines of the prison. What is of concern is that prisoner transportation vehicles, known as 'sweat boxes', are associated with being cramped, claustrophobic and oppressive which is distressing for the prisoner (Caddle, 1995; Howard League, 2001). The prison vehicle is a compartmentalised bus of cells, a human cattle truck, with observation panels, no seat belts, no toilet facilities with the prisoner then urinating in the bag in their 'pod' and an additional dehumanising element. The negative experiences of the prison bus arguably underpin distress prisoners after entry or transfer (Howard League, 2001).

The final pain to be considered is that of *fear or nervousness about release* (Jones, 2007), which is an aggressive stressor for those transferring and transitioning to the open prison estate. In addition to the anxiety and uncertainty stemming from the pains discussed so far, the prisoner moving to the open estate also has to contend with the knowledge that they are in the final stage of their sentence, the penal finishing school if you like – with a range of social interactions and activities to prepare them for release – from where they will be re-integrated into the community. Just as prisoners face elevated stress levels on their entry to prison, they face the same levels of stress on their exit and re-entry into society. Thoughts about problems finding employment, how they will maintain, develop and reconnect family ties alongside how they will fit back into the social world all become products of a heightened anxiety leading up to release (Parisi, 1982; Paulus & Dzindolet, 1992). Thus, the final stages of imprisonment can be fraught with difficulty, which further distorts prisoners' experience of imprisonment and assaults their sense of place, identity and mental health.

Tightness

It is important, therefore, to conceptualise and delineate the pains of imprisonment described in this chapter from other varieties of the penal experience in order to capture the essence of and difference between them. Arguably, the most appropriate term to characterise the experience of imprisonment, certainly in the context of the open prison estate, is that of 'tightness'. In this conceptualisation, institutional power is experienced as a constricting force that envelopes the prisoner subjected to it and one that fuels the prisoner to behave and act in a way that is welcomed by the institution. Crewe (2011a, p. 522) describes this power as working as an 'invisible harness', recognising its elusive yet looming presence, which underpins self-regulation of the prisoner with this application of power. Alford (2000, p. 140) muses that '[t]he ruler still rules, but he rules underground' and astutely observes that 'moved to the margins and rendered more invisible, power has not therefore become more subtle'. This is arguably the case when considering the reconfiguration of power in the prison system. This tightness is evident in this context through the psychological assessment, risk assessment and responsibilisation described and the accountability that it brings. As such, these maintain a vice-like hold over prisoners, reducing them 'to instruments of wilful, omnipresent, and all-pervading force: power' (Franke, 1995, p. 294). In the open prison estate, as discussed, there are a range of very pertinent aspects resulting in pain. The conditions of the open prison, which demand self-regulation due to low levels of staffing and minimal security alongside the 'end stage' of the prisoner's sentence, mean that tightness has a deep entanglement with the fear and insecurity that prisoners have of transitioning to different penal status, to that of an ex-prisoner being released or being returned to a higher security prison. These negative dimensions of tight forms of power are revealed when prisoners fail to subject themselves to the level required by the institution in relation to rules, regulations and self-discipline. The tightness looms over them, waiting in the wings as a form of hard power that ring-fences the purported softer strategy and construction of the open prison.

Crewe and Ievins (2020, p. 3) further argue that this tightness therefore induces prisoners, who are subjected to a 'disciplinary gaze', to exercise self-control from the conditions of autonomy and freedom in the prison. Open prisons are 'loose and lax', as well as 'tight', with both soft and at times, hard power in play. Embedded within a system fraught with deficiency and inconsistency, such a toxic combination continues to have a detrimental impact on those subjected to it. The methods of delivering pain have changed in location from physical to psychological; however, the power has not. As Alford (2000, p. 139) argues, 'prisons [. . .] represent not pain that originates at the margins, but power that has been moved to the margins from the centre, whilst losing none of its centrality'.

Power is Still Power

> Stress is an important feature of prison life, and indeed may be the central feature of prison life as it is experienced by prisoners themselves. Stress can contaminate programs, undermine adjustment efforts, and leave a residue or bitterness and resentment among inmates. It can make prison a destructive and destabilising institution; to ignore stress is to relegate prisons to the business of warehousing spoiled (and spoiling) human resources. Stress must be controlled if prisons are to

> become environments in which the work of corrections, in any sense of the word, can take place. (Johnson & Toch, 1982, p. 20)

Although almost 70 years old, Sykes' work has provided the blueprint for an appreciation and understanding of the pain associated with prisoner experiences of imprisonment. While applicable to a range of contexts, it remained nonetheless narrow in its reach and has now been extended to address a range of other pains associated with imprisonment, indicative of the evolution of the prison to what we know today. Power in prison is experienced as less heavy and hard than it was historically and as much less authoritarian in nature yet these newer pains contribute to imprisonment across the open estate as being 'tight', with the 'soft' psychological power wielded over prisoners, leaving them feeling as though they are in a state of perpetual uncertainty. It is 'at the psychological level that imprisonment is a painful, depriving and destructive experience' (Morris & Morris, 1963, p. 183). Being imprisoned is less directly and overtly oppressive, but more vice-like. The prison is an institution that is still synonymous with pain. In fact, as the system has evolved, it has contributed to the creation and exacerbation of a wider range of pain for those within it and suggests that Johnson and Toch's (1982) warning has not been observed. Pain has not been eliminated in the prison of today. Rather, it has merely morphed into a different construction that attacks the prisoner in a different way to its predecessors. Those who do not adjust easily to these pains are likely to find imprisonment a difficult experience. Johnson and Toch (1982) also state that sometimes the destructive process emanating from the pain of imprisonment occurs in the presence of peers and authorities who choose to do their own time and ignore the suffering and humanity that surround them. The current state of our prisons today demonstrating record levels of self-harm and suicide offers the starkest illustration of these relationships.

Prisoners' Lives Matter

The Department of Health report *Closing the Gap* (2014, p. 4) professes that:

> Mental health is moving up the policy agenda across government. Working together to improve outcomes for people with mental health problems is, therefore, a major policy priority.

It would be interesting to see upon what rung mental health rests on the policy ladder. The evidence presented suggests that it is neither climbing that ladder fast enough nor effectively. Each critical juncture and report call for a greater awareness of the issues in our prisons, but this should have always been an important consideration. If it had, then there would be no need for the consistent report recommendations for it to be so. Perhaps it is that the level of policy importance hinges on the intricate interplay between public attitudes and sentiment towards punishment, imprisonment and the political climate. After all, the focus and developments charted in relation to the mental health of prisoners, and indeed prisons themselves, either stem from or rely upon the mobilisation of public opinion. As Bradley (2009, p. 9) asserts, '[t]he issues may remain the same, but what has changed over the intervening years is the political and social context'. There is a pattern that pervades this entire era of penal work. A range of harmful enduring penal issues metastasise throughout the penal system in England and Wales. These issues may have differed in their construction, severity and extent and been subject to several reformatory processes with variability in success, yet the fact remains that they are consistently present and, by their very nature, continue to have detrimental effects on prisoners. Prisons are under increasing pressure, making it more challenging to manage prisoner mental health and well-being. Reduced resources, restricted regimes and outdated and ageing facilities all affect mental health and well-being in custodial settings. These issues arguably culminate in immense distress for prisoners synonymous with the 'corrosive nature of imprisonment' (Liebling, 1999). Bradley (2009, p. 9) perhaps expresses best the position evidenced regarding mental health in the England and Wales penal system when he notes that '[it] is hard to believe that what was relevant [...] years ago is just as relevant today and that we are still struggling to resolve the same problems'.

While these reports recognise conditions and dynamics in prison that underpin the poor mental health and well-being of those imprisoned, it is key to acknowledge that what has been introduced to address these has not worked. The charted efforts that have been previously made to genuinely improve outcomes relating to suicide prevention, safety and decency are being eroded by austere conditions (Crewe & Liebling, 2017). However, just like the Gladstone Committee were not deterred by the issues the prison system was besieged by many criminal justice actors have not either. As such, there has been a continued quest to improve the condition of our prisons and issues they face as well as the mental health and well-being outcomes for the prison population. The reports covered in this chapter are a foundation for new approaches in the next stage of reform.

The evolution of contemporary penal practices, such as power-sharing initiatives which are symbolic of reconfigured penal power, are steeped in the assumption that 'power in prison is inherently bad' (Crewe et al., 2014, p. 8). They have often been viewed from a perspective riddled with scepticism and the perception that they are sinister in nature and 'involving [...] repression, domination and subjection' (McMahon, 1992, p. 218). This outlook has often served to preclude the fact that coercion is merely one aspect of power relations in prison and is not its essence. Good power, utilised with the intent to produce positive quality of life, safety and other custodial custody outcomes through power-sharing initiatives – such as the use of peer support schemes and programmes in custodial settings – can achieve positive outcomes. Current safer custody strategies recognise the importance of peer supporters in the custodial environment, with peer support becoming an increasingly prominent facet in the promotion of health and well-being and instrumental in reducing suicide and self-harm in custody, as well as supporting the mental health issues of the prison population, through providing support to other prisoners in situations that could trigger distress (Davies, 1994; Snow & Biggar, 2006; Woodall et al., 2015).

In recent times, there has been a clamour for more innovative and progressive intervention across the prison estate, with one of the most recent advances centring around the re-configuration of penal power, with power-sharing initiatives between staff and prisoners being employed to 'bridge the gap' and produce better offender outcomes, especially in relation to mental health through 'peer support'. The next chapter explores peer support in the context of imprisonment.

Chapter 3

'Pain Management': Peer Support in Prison

A significant public health concern is the pronounced health disparities experienced by those imprisoned in comparison to those in the community (Sturup-Toft et al., 2018; Walton et al., 2023, 2025). As established in the preceding chapters, those imprisoned exhibit significantly elevated rates of mental health disorders compared to those in the general population, and there is an intensification during imprisonment (McLeod et al., 2020; PRI, 2022; Sturup-Toft et al., 2018; Walton et al., 2025). These issues frequently manifest as substance abuse, self-harm and suicide (Baybutt et al., 2019; Fazel et al., 2011). Given these health disparities, it is imperative to ensure that those imprisoned receive adequate care for their mental health needs; however, prison environments encounter persistent issues of overcrowding, insufficient staffing, inadequate financing and security and operational limitations (Fletcher & Batty, 2012; Walton et al., 2025).

There is currently the realisation among policymakers that such issues compromise engagement with statutory services (Scott & Codd, 2010). As such, a culture of 'doing more' has pervaded penal institutions, arising from the combination of increasingly austere prison conditions and the potential of power-sharing initiatives to produce positive outcomes on prisoner mental health and well-being. With establishments seeking to bridge the gap between staff and their institutions on one side of the divide and offenders on the other, using prisoner peer support workers and initiatives to deliver positive outcomes – as well as stretch their limited resources further – there is often the mandate to do not just more but more with less (Fletcher & Batty, 2012).

Peer support is becoming an increasingly important component of the promotion of health and well-being, and current safer custody policies recognise its value in the custodial setting. It has been shown to play a significant role in lowering the rate of suicide and self-harm and aiding the population of prisoners who have mental health conditions (Davies, 1994; Perrin, 2024; Snow & Biggar, 2006; Woodall et al., 2015). Despite variations in their typologies, they all share the premise that, in prison settings, they are recognised as being programmes for prisoners by prisoners (Ehly & Vazquez, 1998; Kerish, 1975). In such settings, induction-related peer support schemes are often delivered by Induction Insiders or Induction Peer Support Workers. Inducting prisoners to the policy, procedures

Navigating Mental Health in the Male Open Prison, 43–59

doi:10.1108/978-1-83549-706-720251003

and day-to-day lived regime of the prison establishment while providing reassurance and practical support to prisoners has become a prominent aspect of peer support in the early days after their arrival at the new establishment. The experiential knowledge of prisoner peers can legitimise, amplify and give credence to communication and action by prison staff, which is often rebuffed or lacking impact in the eyes of those imprisoned.

Despite the explosion of peer interventions across the prison estate, illustrated by 7% of prisoners said to be involved as peer supporters across England and Wales, there is a lack of large-scale studies of them (Jarrett, 2018) with the sparse research that does exist being narrow, compartmentalised and 'largely functional, aiming to evidence reduced reoffending rates' (Buck, 2018, p. 191). It does so at the expense of focusing on the nuanced aspect of these interventions in differing contexts and how they work to influence change in those exposed to them.

This chapter firstly establishes the notion of peer intervention, introduces the differing typologies of peer education, peer mentoring and peer support that exist and reconciles them to provide a working definition of peer intervention within the penal estate. The chapter then moves on to consider the roots of peer intervention and its development institutionally, from its early use in healthcare, educational and youth service settings to its rise as an ever-present feature of the penal estate across England and Wales. In doing so, it considers the development of penal intervention, especially in the realm of offending behaviour, which has paved the way for a wider range of interventions. It also establishes a shift in ethos, from prisoners being seen as passive recipient in the penal institution to an active institutional resource.

The chapter then considers the theoretical underpinnings of peer intervention and peer induction specifically an entanglement of differing aspects of Social Learning Theory, Social Inoculation Theory and Differential Association Theory. It is these theoretical positions that are invariably drawn on to inform the design and implementation of peer intervention. Being such a prominent yet diffuse concept, power is considered in the context of peer intervention, considering power as a positive force in custodial settings and that peer-led induction contains a number of power relations that ultimately provide a level of social support. It is this that acts as a 'buffer' from the challenges and difficulties that mentees face and specifically those in the adaptation to a new prison setting. The chapter moves on to then look at peer interventions in practise in penal settings, focusing on two prominent endeavours representing passive and active models of peer support. Ultimately, peer intervention is about delivering beneficial outcomes, and the chapter considers research into the efficacy of peer intervention in prisons. In doing so, it considers the benefits of peer interventions both for individuals and the institution while also identifying and considering a range of issues that reveal a fragile underbelly to peer support that both challenges and threatens the effectiveness of such interventions.

Peer Interventions

There is a breadth of constructs of, and terminologies for, peer interventions and peer workers in custodial settings. Peer mentor, peer educator, peer listener, peer supporter and peer counsellor are frequently used terms for workers of interventions of those principles and are often used interchangeably without recognition of their differences. Collectively, peer interventions are described as 'complex interventions as there are typically a number of inter-related components both in relation to the preparation, training and supervision of peer workers and in relation to their subsequent role and interactions with the target population' (Woodall et al., 2015, p. 7). It is, in fact, difficult to delineate these completely as there is significant overlap between them, and arguably, elements of all can exist within an intervention. As such, there has been significant difficulty in finding a singular encompassing definition of peer intervention with it being 'widely acknowledged that no one single definition or model exists, rather a number of different models providing support' (Parsons et al., 2008, p. 5). It is important therefore, at this juncture, to provide an overview of the three key categories of peer interventions within the prison system to care.

Peer education is predominately focused on the provision of communication, education and skill development, which is an endeavour between prisoners with the desired outcome to increase knowledge and awareness and to influence change in the recipient. Peer education is typically associated with health promotion and harm reduction surrounding HIV/AIDS, sexual health and injecting practices, with the peer educators having undergone training in the knowledge base and skill to deliver education to the audience.

Peer mentoring involves establishing a relationship between two individuals, the mentor typically acting as a role model or experiential authority figure who has successfully navigated the path the mentee will soon take and who supports the development of the mentee. In the prison environment, this relationship is often related to goals surrounding effective resettlement, social inclusion and desistance (Joliffe & Farrington, 2007). However, research has identified mentoring interventions as also improving mental health outcomes (Perrin, 2017). As well as reinforcing positive attitudes and behaviours, interventions often introduce instrumental support.

Peer support in prisons involves either social, emotional or practical support being provided by peer support workers. Peer support interventions can involve group work or can alternatively be one-to-one, dependent on identified prisoner needs. This support can take the form of counselling, listening, befriending, liaison with staff and providing information and signposting (Perrin, 2017). Peer support involves the provision of emotional support to the recipient to allow them to release the stress that they had accumulated. Examples include the Listeners Scheme, a prison suicide prevention scheme present throughout the prison estate and linked to the Samaritans, and the Insiders Scheme, an induction programme for new prisoners entering a custodial establishment. The latter is indicative of this with peer supporters offered elements of 'reassurance, information and practical assistance…to new prisoners'. (Perrin, 2017, p. 13) although it is not necessarily intended to provide emotional support.

Prison Service Instruction (PSI) offers instructions on peer support as outlined in PSI 17/2015 (NOMS, 2015). This PSI was created to offer guidelines on peer support programs in penal settings. The PSI asserts that peer support must adhere to explicit and uniform rules, establishing distinct boundaries about the prisoner's role to ensure the protection of both the peer supporter and the individual receiving support. The essential criteria for general peer support are delineated below. The stipulations outlined in the PSI pertain to five principal areas: (1) training and oversight, (2) boundaries, (3) explicit employment procedures, (4) collaborative engagement and (5) evaluation. Another pertinent PSI regarding peer support schemes pertains to adult safeguarding in prisons is PSI 16/2015 (NOMS, 2015), which underscores the obligation of prisons to safeguard adult inmates from various forms of abuse (including physical, emotional and institutional) and neglect (see Fig. 1 summary).

This overview provides a scaffold to distinguish the differing characteristics of peer intervention models and also their areas of overlap. To reflect the entanglement of some of these characteristics and programmes, this chapter refers to them under the umbrella term of peer support interventions and draws upon a working definition as involving 'the provision of education, support or counselling between individuals who are of equal social status or who share similar characteristics or who have common experiences' (Woodall et al., 2015). In the context of peer-led induction, those prisoners involved in the delivery of the intervention are referred to as peer support workers from herein, to reflect these entangled characteristics in a peer-led induction. It is to the starting point of peer support that this chapter now turns as it charts the roots and evolution of penal and peer intervention.

History and Development of Peer-Based Intervention

Programmes and interventions in the contemporary prison have historically been directed at eliciting a reduction in re-offending through some form of positive change. This can be social change through welfare provision or at the individual level (Hollin & Palmer, 2006). This rehabilitative ideal, however, was sharply experienced during the 1980s alongside the marked move to the right and the shift to a 'just deserts' model of administration to those coming into contact with the criminal justice system. This stemmed from a 'nothing works' perspective, with rehabilitative measures seemingly having no effect on recidivism (Lipton et al., 1975). Eliminative measures used at the time, such as short sharp shock prison regimes, were illustrative of this gravitation to more punitive measures. Questions continued to rise about what could be done to rehabilitate prisoners effectively to prevent crime and reduce re-offending. What the analyses were able to garner were factors for effective offender interventions. These may be cognitive behavioural in nature, structured programmes with specific aims an objective, an elevated level of treatment integrity, delivery by highly trained staff, with prominent levels of organisational support, and built in monitoring and

Prison Service Instruction	General peer support or social care specific?	Topic PSI relates to
• The benefits of peer support must be explained to peers (mandatory)	General	Training
• Peers must not be relied on to provide care that is the responsibility of health and social care providers (mandatory)	General	Boundaries
• Peers and recipients must be made aware of the limits of peer support (i.e. what they are and are not allowed to do), and that these boundaries must be explained in a care plan (or if not, recorded locally) (mandatory)	General	Training, boundaries and monitoring
• Peers must be appropriately selected, risk assessed, trained, supported and supervised (mandatory)	General	Employment processes, training and supervision
• Peer support schemes should be formal arrangements in which peers are paid for their work or aware that they are acting as unpaid volunteers (mandatory)	General	Employment processes
• Peers and recipients must know of safeguarding policies and how to raise concerns should abuse or neglect arise (mandatory)	General	Training
• Peer support schemes may be supported by partner organisations but remain the responsibility of the prison (mandatory)	General	Collaborative working

Fig. 1. PSI and Peer Support. *Source:* Walton et al. (2025).

evaluation procedures (Hollin & Palmer, 2006, p. 4). These principles provide a strong guiding set for the development and implementation of interventions and, as Hollin and Palmer (2006, p. 6) assert, 'provide a basis from which to extend theory, research and practice'. Interventions in prison in the 1990s gained momentum, underpinned by a clearer notion of what worked, and there was now a further focus to ensure action spoke louder than words. Programmes had to demonstrate they employed these principles and that the quality of delivery was high. The answer to ensuring high-quality intervention and delivery integrity was through accreditation and audit. Until 2006, the Correctional Services Accreditation Panel has evidenced 'no shortage of well-developed, accredited programmes in the Prison and Probation Services of England and Wales' (Hollin & Palmer, 2006, p. 19) and in the years since 1999 has 'accredited 27 offending behaviour programmes, recognised or provisionally accredited four programmes, one integrated system, and a model for a prison therapeutic community' (Hollin & Palmer, 2006, p. 19).

Despite the focus on offending behaviour and programmes that target specific offenders or offences, within a dominant discourse and relentless targeting of re-offending, many of the principles discussed have been used as the foundation for wider ranges of interventions in prison, interventions delivering awareness, education and support existing outside of the recidivism vacuum. These have some constructionist values, and such approaches involve employing education, skill training, employability skills and intervention to change attitudes and beliefs and equip offenders with skills to navigate life. Although they often seek to change criminal behaviour through providing alternatives to offending, they also have impact to bring about many positive outcomes further afield in the individual rather than being contained purely in relation to re-offending and criminal behaviour. Peer support interventions and indeed peer-led induction are primary examples of these.

Peer support as an element of interventions and programmes is evident as early as 1793 in clinical settings for those with mental illness, with peers seen as better suited to that work because of their honesty and humanity (Davidson et al., 2012). Miller and MacGilchrist (1996) and Parkin and McKeganey (2000) have traced the roots of peer education to education settings in 19th century England with pupils assisting teachers with lessons. It was from the 1920s when a focus on the value on the role of peer support in the treatment of mental disorders was applied (Davidson et al., 2012). In an inpatient facility for male schizophrenics, men recovering from mental health issues were enlisted by the medical personnel to assist on a treatment unit. Personnel were firmly of the belief that the combination of their own life experiences of their mental health issues and recovery would add a dimension to their work, making them uniquely qualified to 'assist their peers in working through similar struggles in a humane and compassionate manner' (Davidson et al., 2012, p. 3).

This approach paved the way for the operation of many therapeutic and clinical settings in the years since. Subsequent therapeutic communities developed in inpatient settings have encouraged the use of peer support and mentoring, as well as 'confrontation, conflict, and collaborative problem-solving', as integral elements of the treatment process (Davidson et al., 2012, p. 6). In contemporary times, peer interventions have migrated from their primary usage in healthcare settings and have been largely associated with use within educational and youth service settings such as schools, with these interventions targeting a range of issues largely associated with social welfare such as sex education, learning difficulties, drug consumption, substance abuse, anger management and violence. Studies into the peer support interventions in these realms share the perspective that outcomes from these interventions are positive (Devilly et al., 2005; Fletcher & Batty, 2012; Shiner, 1999; South et al., 2014; Walton et al., 2025). The common themes that exist across the schemes, irrespective of the variance in their design, is their foundations on the core values of mutual reciprocity, shared problem-solving, empathy and experiential exchange (Blagden & Perrin, 2014).

There is a basic understanding of peer support as being the embodiment of these values. The sharing of experience and learning from those like 'us' is founded upon them, yet it is a complex proposition. This complexity starts from the contention of what or who a peer is; close friends, associates, other people in a shared environment or task could all be described as peers. However, as Shiner (1999, p. 557) postulates, 'the question remains, what makes somebody like us?' In short, identity. Individuals construct and mould identities in relation to an array of characteristics, which can emanate from a range of sources. Shiner (1999) advances that these can include roles that social actors take on, group categories they feel attached to and experiences that they have. In the prison environment, a peer can be identified through being someone who belongs to the same group category of the mentee, namely a prisoner, and who has the same experiences of prison, more specifically the experiences and challenges that the mentee will be experiencing. However, this is a broad construction.

As such, there is the potential for identity conflicts, with tensions arising from other characteristics of the peer such as ethnicity, race, sexual orientation and more prison specific notions such as offence type, sentence type and the affiliation with those in power. There is a multitude of outcomes, some good, some unintended and some not necessarily positive that may emerge given the complexities involved in a multiplicity of dimensions to identity. All can undermine relationships with mentees and peer support workers and, ultimately, the intervention. Historically, those imprisoned were recognised as passive recipients of treatment who to adopted the role of patient or client, with professional staff being the active agents (Devilly et al., 2005). However, it has long been established in the realm of counsellor preferences in the penal estate that clients 'prefer one of their own kind' (Cahill et al., 1979). The idea that prisoners provide social support to one another during their day-to-day prison life has been identified as an informal mechanism in many accounts of imprisonment (Sykes, 1958).

Considering this, it is important to return to the idea that peer-led induction is an example of re-configured penal power. The intervention is illustrative of the shift from those associated with the structures of authority, namely prison staff, doing induction, to prisoners being enabled to lead and deliver the intervention. In doing so, it recognises prisoners as moving beyond passive recipients of intervention to being 'important resources' (Boothby, 2011, p. 426) in the support of prisoners. Given the shifts in penal power in the contemporary prison, rather than being recipients, prisoners are now identified as a legitimised resource, with the formal capacity to both powerfully and positively influence their peers (Devilly et al., 2005; McHugh, 1995). As such, they have been identified as having the potential to facilitate a closing of the gulf between what is needed and what is provided (Fletcher & Batty, 2012).

Though social support has been conceptualised in a number of ways, there is agreement that it relates to an exchange of resources between individuals. Exchanges are by nature two-way, which means that a person may either give or receive. Peer initiatives are sometimes referred to as an internal social support system that comes from within the institution. It can be formal when its source has official status, such as the criminal justice system, and informal when emanating from one of the recipients' social connections (Boothby, 2011; Cullen, 1994). Peer-led induction transcends across both realms in its operation, with the overall outcome being that internal formal support has demonstrated the ability to increase the quality of prison life and support prisoners to navigate the prison environment (Boothby, 2011; Ryan & McCabe, 1994).

When explaining the role of social support on well-being, the Buffering Model is arguably the most pertinent theoretical basis. Emerging from the field of medicine, the theory argues that people who receive social support are able to better cope in situations of illness or other physical ailment and benefit from an increased sense of well-being (Lo, 2019). It advances that social support has a significant positive effect when individuals are under high stress and that when social support is high, individuals will develop fewer psychological problems. Given that transfer and adaptation to a new prison establishment are identified triggers of mental health issues and manifestations in the form of self-harm and suicide, peer-led induction arguably works as a form of buffering as it seeks to redefine the threat of a situation and maximise the ability of the individual to cope with it. Again, this theory does not sit in isolation, as some individuals may not experience heightened psychological effects stemming from transfer and transition, and as such, it is important to also consider the more generalised idea of the Main Effect Model. This rather contends that social support has a positive effect on well-being in both high and low states of stress (Boothby, 2011; Cohen & Wills, 1985). While peer-led induction is not intended to be a dedicated emotional support, it nonetheless incorporates notions of emotional support alongside being a source of practical support and information, emphasising the importance of this as a social support system, irrespective of whether it buffers in situations of high stress or regardless of the level of stress.

Returning to the notion of peer support as a resource, this word is employed given that, rather than be a purely humanistic endeavour to promote the best possible outcomes for those experiencing it, it has a more dominant fiscal underbelly for the institution. With re-offending costing upwards of £13 billion (National Audit Office, 2010), it should perhaps come as no surprise that the quest for new and innovative ways to address offending behaviour are at the forefront of criminal justice policy. Fletcher and Batty (2012, p. 14) home in on the notion of public spending cuts meaning that there is a shift on focus to 'doing more with less'. This arguably arises given the continued austerity measures that pervade the public sector. Peer support is a cost-effective intervention, with the use of peers considerably cheaper than prison staff.

Prison Peer Intervention in Practice

There are many ways that prisoners are involved in peer interventions across the England and Wales prisons estate: Health Trainers, Resettlement Champions, Recovery Champions, Prison Council Representatives, Shannon Trust Mentors, Heath Care Representatives and the St, Giles Trust Advice Project are just some of the many interventions and roles that are present in prisons, demonstrating the breadth across the different areas of imprisonment. A summary of some of the most common prison-based schemes that involve peers can be seen in Table 2.

There are predominately two models of such peer interventions in prisons. The first being that peer support is seen as a passive intervention such as the Samaritans' Listeners Scheme whereas peer-led induction is viewed as being active in nature with the characteristics of providing advice and help (Fletcher & Batty, 2012). Considering these two interventions, illustrative of these models to draw out the differences in approach is important at this juncture as they are divergent in achieving their intended outcomes.

Table 2. Peer Support Schemes in Prisons in England and Wales.

Scheme Title	Nature of Support	Description
Listeners	Emotional	Volunteer Listeners who are trained by the external charity Samaritans provide face-to-face emotional support to prisoners who request help.
Buddies	Emotional and practical	Buddies can be paired with new prisoners who may require emotional support and also practical assistance when first adjusting to life in [a new] prison.
Helping Hands	Personal care	Helping Hands volunteers care for those less able to do so for themselves. This role can involve personal care duties as well as emotional and practical support.
Shannon Trust Mentors	Educational	The Shannon Trust is a UK charity that regulates a scheme within which fluent readers are paired with those less able. Through this set-up, mentors help students through a reading programme over a period of several months.

Source: Perrin (2019, pp. 6–7).

There is no better place to start than with the most prominent intervention, a passive one, the Listeners Scheme. First launched in HMP Swansea in 1991, it is now a scheme available in almost every prison in England and Wales. The intervention is described by the Samaritans as a 'a peer support service which aims to reduce suicide and self-harm in prisons' (The Samaritans, 2022). These listeners provide a confidential service in the form of emotional passive support to their peers who are experiencing difficulties coping in prison. They are trained by the Samaritans and sign a code of conduct with them. These listeners have supervision regularly and attend safer custody meetings within the prison, indicative of their role in improving safer custody outcomes for those that they engage with. Prisoners who are experiencing emotional distress can access this provision by calling out listeners who meet with them in a dedicated area in the prison. One of its main characteristics is that it demands confidentiality, and this is an element that makes it more accessible for those needing help and who may have been otherwise reluctant to seek it (Scowcroft et al., 2019). Passive schemes such as the Listeners do lack the dynamism and depth of more active interventions and therefore are limited in the support they can provide, especially in context-fluid situations. Also there exist concerns about how 'confidential' such a service can be in the prison environment from when there is a level of both prisoner and staff involvement in the provision of the service.

The most pertinent peer support intervention in prisons across England and Wales, certainly of relevance to this book, is the Insiders Scheme, an active form of peer intervention, and more specifically, induction-based peer support. The Insiders Scheme was conceived as an active form of engagement to target the initial prison experience of prisoners which is synonymous with elevated levels of self-harm and suicide. In fact, the first 24 hours and first week in prison are associated with the highest risk of suicidal behaviour in prisoners. They are also recognised as 'high risk periods for establishing harmful relationships with staff and prisoners' (Adair, 2005), which also signifies the interaction between relationships and potential deficiencies in the experience of imprisonment. It is an intervention that has concurrent objectives of reducing anxiety experienced in the early days of custody and improving safer custody outcomes. The scheme operates as a multifaceted endeavour, comprising differing elements. Prisoners, who work as 'Insiders', are more active in their role and have more scope than those carrying out passive support. As such, they are described as being more 'advice and practicality orientated rather than listening and emotion focussed' (Perrin, 2017, p. 26) in offering information and reassurance to help new prisoners navigate these stressful early days in custody and the challenges of adaptation, following their arrival at an establishment. This advice and support can be in relation to Offender Management, Family Support, Chaplaincy, Steroid Information, Resettlement, Safer Custody, Education Assessment, Working Out Scheme, Drug and Alcohol Support (RAPT), Independent Monitoring Board and Gym Awareness. Peers will often use a checklist to ensure that all the relevant aspects of their role have been delivered. These are then signed by the prisoner mentee to signify that they have received and understood the relevant information, and they can take it with them after induction. Peer support workers are usually selected by the frontline staff working on reception, first-night and induction and then subjected to security clearance by the prison.

Selection criteria for peer support workers can include the type of offence, as well as those prisoners having no history of bullying and no recent failed drug tests. It is suggested that they be trustworthy, literate, caring and good communicators with appropriate interpersonal skills. They are traditionally supervised by staff involved in the reception and induction process and those staff should advise and support them also. Senior Management Team (SMT) and prison staff backing is noted as a core component of such schemes being fully effective. The schemes also require open and honest communication with the staff involved and balance between the benefits and potential drawbacks, such as fears of scheme abuse and conflicts with the security of the establishment. Some of these peer support roles are voluntary while others are paid positions; again, this is dependent on the individual prison. The key focus is that peers lead induction delivery and feed into the process, supporting the staff who are involved.

Despite there being caution raised about peer mentoring and peer support being used interchangeably and their nuanced differences in relation to being passive or active, there is nonetheless the reality that often elements of both approaches are combined and overlap and that certainly appears to be the case in relation to peer induction.

Theoretical Underpinnings of Prison Peer Support Interventions

Tolan et al. (2008) advance pillars of mentoring applicable to prison-based peer intervention more generally, yet there are three of those relating directly to peer-led induction. Firstly, peer-to-peer work should involve interaction between two individuals. Secondly, the mentor in the relationship holds and evidences a level of experience, knowledge or power that is greater than the mentee, with this construction of power much aligned with the behaviourist models of peer support which will be discussed later in the chapter. Thirdly, the mentee should be able to benefit from the knowledge, skills and experience of the mentor. Buck (2018, p. 192) also proposes that there are three fundamental conditions of peer mentoring, 'caring, listening and encouraging small steps' that a good mentor will demonstrate and manage in the course of their interactions with mentees. Moving away from the cost-effective nature of using peers Fletcher and Batty (2012) also identify a further three key tenets underpinning the use of peer interventions:

(1) Peers are effective identity models and as such they enable the Social Learning and Inoculation Theory.
(2) Use of peers are necessary to mitigate and navigate the view of prison staff as authority figures without first-hand experience.
(3) Peer intervention builds social capital and resilience within a prison community that can be described as one of deprivation and complexity.

When considering peer interventions from a theoretical perspective, these core pillars provide an initial grounding for a more general explanation of how peer support interventions work and also serve as an indication of the enactment and influence of re-configured penal power. In terms of a more specific theoretical explanation, Social Learning Theory, Social Inoculation Theory and Differential Association Theory all demonstrate a combination of elements that predominately underpin peer interventions in custodial settings. While considered separately, it is proposed that some elements are interchangeable, supporting the idea that peer intervention is indicative of a theoretical and thus practical hybrid in the prison.

Firstly, Social Learning Theory commits to the notion that behavioural change among individuals comes from the opportunity to observe and practice behaviours garnered from others until they are able to model them effectively (Turner & Shepherd, 1999). The extent of this influence is determined by the model's qualities, the observer's traits and the perceptions of the results of adhering to such behaviours (Bandura, 1986; Devilly et al., 2005). It acknowledges that many prisoners have both chaotic and complex circumstances that have maligned their learning process, with their developmental curve being founded upon and affected at all junctures by a range of parenting influences and anti-social traits. As such, the opportunity to be exposed to and interact with a range of fellow prisoners demonstrating pro-social attitudes and behaviours, and overcoming similar antecedent circumstances, acts as a form of experiential knowledge exchange between peer mentors and peer mentees (Borkman, 1990) and is an effective method to bring about attitudinal and behavioural change (Devilly et al., 2005; Mathie & Ford, 1998; Turner & Shepherd, 1999).

Secondly, Social Inoculation Theory places emphasis on the social pressures that compromise an individual's resilience to unhealthy attitudes and behaviours. The theory suggests that resistance to such pressure is strengthened by developing arguments to counter them (Turner & Shepherd, 1999). Interventions designed to help develop those counter arguments delivered by professional service staff within the prison can be rejected by prisoners. However, when those counter arguments are delivered by those who share the same lived experiences and pressures, they can land more successfully (Devilly et al., 2005).

Finally, Differential Association Theory (Cressey, 1960) draws upon the psychological concepts of both Social Learning and Inoculation theories but stems from criminological and deviance research. It argues that offending behaviour can be learnt by those interacting with those who can teach the skills and techniques to offend. That is a negative consideration of this, yet conversely, Turner and Shepherd (1999) argue that those acting as peer supporters can also act as the catalyst and facilitator for helping those they interact with to change their behaviour and lifestyles. Moving beyond purely offending behaviour, this theory can be applied to supporting those adapting and transitioning to a new establishment through peer-led induction, with new prisoners learning from interactions with their peers who have walked the same path previously.

While these are broad and generalised theories underpinning the usage and effectiveness of peer support, elements of all theories are arguably present in peer-led induction, albeit to differing levels dependent on the intervention framing, aims and strategies. Certainly, in a peer induction intervention, the presence of all of these theories can be seen to inform the design and implementation of the intervention.

Benefits of Prison Peer-Based Interventions

In the literature that exists, much has been said about the benefits and impact of peer interventions in custodial settings. Current suicide prevention recognises the importance of peer supporters as an increasingly prominent facet in the promotion of health and well-being with clear indications of positive practical and/or emotional effects for the recipients of peer interventions. Those who had used peer support reported using it as an avenue to 'vent and to overcome feelings of anxiety, loneliness, depression and self-injury, and there were indications that this may be potentially beneficial in preventing suicides in prison' (South et al., 2014, p. 47). It is also indicated by South et al. (2014) that there are attitudinal and behaviour improvements among those receiving peer support. Further research identifies peer support as instrumental in supporting increased emotional well-being, the ability to confront offending behaviour, increased social functionality, social inclusion and a reduction in the likelihood of developing a mental disorder or the degree of mental disorder (Davies, 1994; Fletcher & Batty, 2012; Snow & Biggar, 2006; South et al., 2014; Woodall et al., 2015). This, in turn, can underpin elevated safety and better returns on the money spent on imprisonment (World Health Organisation, 1998).

While the use of peer support is implemented, often with the sole and explicit aim of promoting well-being, an increase in power-sharing between staff and prisoners is also evidenced (Crewe & Liebling, 2017, p. 905). With the idea of doing less with more and new and innovative ways of 'doing prison' (navigating prison and sentences) – a prominent concern of the prison service in the face of austerity measures – there is undoubtedly a lot of support for peer support. This is especially true from an operational standpoint, given the benefits of peer support interventions for the organisation. Peer supporting prisoners effectively acts as a diversion service in some interventions, especially that of peer-led induction. Peers are sometimes employed to 'absorb queries and issues that would otherwise be directed at prison staff' (Woodall et al., 2015). By default, this allows the time of professional staff to be deployed in other areas of the prison and to other duties in their role. This can be deemed a 'selling point' to garner management buy in to the implementation of peer interventions. Freeing up staff time can arguably help them meet their targets, a prominent cog in the penal wheel. The impact on reducing staff workload is also associated with reducing staff turnover and that it is more cost effective (Boyce et al., 2009; Cook et al., 2008). Given the meagre wages that prisoners are paid, the opportunity to have a workforce available 24 hours a day and 7 days a week makes the ability to run such interventions more financially viable and enhances the productivity of the prison workforce.

Peers primarily are seen as credible individuals to engage with the target audience. This is extremely important in the role of peer induction interventions as they are seen as 'more credible sources of information [who have] experienced similar struggles and [...] speak the same language by offering positive support and positive role modelling' (Devilly et al., 2005, p. 232). As such, in prison, mentees are deemed more likely to turn to peers than authority figures and those associated with the structures of power. Peers with this credibility are effective at sharing information and knowledge, the founding principles of a peer-led induction intervention. In fact, it is evidenced that individuals are more inclined to be receptive to this information when it is presented to them by someone they can identify with. Also, given their knowledge of the prison context and environment, peers themselves can better engage in a manner that most effectively conveys information (Fletcher & Batty, 2012). The benefits of credibility also extend into the running of the prison with the use of peers to overcome prisoner issues and challenges, as well as helping prison staff deal with those whose behaviour they find challenging, thereby helping to promote the security and order of the prison establishment.

Risks and Challenges of Prison-Based Peer Interventions

> An appropriately designed and supported peer-led program can have [...] positive effects, expressed in enhanced prisoner wellbeing, reduced rates of self-harm and a calmer and more cooperative social environment. (Adair, 2005, p. 13)

The efficacy of peer-led intervention, specifically induction, is not disputed. The evidence of this is documented in this very chapter. However, what happens when its design and level of support is not appropriate? What does a peer-led induction look like then? It is argued that despite the plentiful beneficial impacts of peer support in the prison environment, research indicates that peer interventions can create a range of negative individual and organisational effects. It is therefore important now to consider these.

Much of the success of any peer intervention within prisons rests on the relationship between staff and peers sharing power. Prisoners do not deliver peer support alone and such interventions invariably require 'buy in' from prison staff, something that South et al. (2014, p. 107) term 'Co-Constructs'. This starts at senior management level, whose support signals the institutional buy in to such interventions. Yet, as this trickles down there remains a requirement for buy in from the boots on the floor. Woodall et al. (2015) advance that those staff who are fully versed with the reasoning for and benefits of peer intervention underpin more successful interventions. However, resistance to interventions compromises facilitation, delivery and ultimate effectiveness and those prison staff resisting can do so logistically by impeding movement of peers or act like 'street level bureaucrats', resisting policy implementation and subvert it (Lipsky, 1969). In fact, the shift in power produced by bestowing more autonomy on prisoners is viewed by some staff as being contentious and problem laden. For example, at an organisational level the idea of allowing prisoners a greater degree of freedom and movement in prison is difficult to overcome and that this actively goes against the grain of prison values, especially among staff cultures and viewpoints about a prisoner being subordinate. Another concern revolves around the use of peers as a 'managerial strategy' to replace paid staff (Woodall et al., 2015). As already introduced, there has become a culture in prisons of doing less with more in the face of austere measures, so there may be a perception among staff that peers are replacements for staff in light of staff redundancies and other cost cutting measures. These can all contrive to underpin staff resistance to peer support.

Confidentiality also remains a key consideration in peer support. Whereas some interventions hold confidentiality as a key tenet, such as the Listeners Scheme, other schemes, including The Induction Insiders, are not a confidential endeavour. There is a strong presence of an inmate code in prison which has various informal rules, including not informing on prisoners to prison staff or those in authority. However, staff may well pressure mentors to disclose and inform on prisoner mentees, and, furthermore, prisoner mentors may well do so for personal gain or to 'settle scores' with prisoners who they may have a slight with (Fletcher & Batty, 2012). Prisoners can fear that disclosing personal information at a time of vulnerability could be used to blackmail, extort or manipulate them when they arrive on their wing. This potential abuse of trust means that peer mentees may in fact gravitate away from a peer-led intervention and towards talking instead to prison staff (Delveaux & Blanchete, 2000). Irrespective of reasoning for it, a lack of confidentiality may certainly affect the application of an induction peer intervention as mentees may naturally, in their heightened state in the early days of custody, view induction staff and mentors through a narrow and wary lens, unwilling to fully immerse into such an intervention to gain from it fully. Linked closely to this notion is the recruitment of those prisoners to be mentors who have the appropriate level of 'experience, aptitude and skill' (Fletcher & Batty, 2012, p. 7). Finding those with those skills and emotional maturity from a population beset by profound complexity in their identity is difficult. As such, there is the potential for the wrong mix of peers to be employed in the face of satisfying demand for peers to facilitate an intervention. Conversely, restricting access to peer supporter positions for those not meeting the criteria required may also preclude those who would potentially make a difference in the role.

In prisons, there has been a long-standing debate about whether they are places of care or control and whether they can manage these dual aims. There exists the reality that institutional concerns about security and order are too dominant over the notions of care, fairness and dignity of those imprisoned. Security concerns are seemingly at the forefront of those involved in the prison system, with discourse being prominent surrounding peer interventions potentially jeopardising security measures in prisons as well as the safe running of the prison. Seemingly, these are based on risk averseness regarding peer workers abusing their positions of power and trust. There are recorded instances of security breaches leading to peer dismissals, such as failed drug tests, the distribution of contraband around the prison, extortion and bullying (Boyce et al., 2009; Fletcher & Batty, 2012; Woodall et al., 2015). Following on from this is the idea that such complexity in peer interventions requires demands on time and labour (Walker & Avis, 1999) that simply aren't available given that interventions, especially induction interventions, have one eye on extending sparse resources by utilising peers in the first place. Prison populations are widely decreed as being difficult to manage, largely predicated by the complex circumstances of those within the penal system, so managing members of these populations as a workforce brings additional challenges which, in turn, constrains resources.

One such issue undermining peer intervention and especially induction is that of peer turnover. The prison population is widely acknowledged as being transient in nature. Prison transfers for a variety of reasons such as progression and disciplinary reasons means that the continuity and effectiveness of interventions can be diminished by attrition among the peer workforce (Scott et al., 2004). This is especially difficult, given that peers are often trained in these specialised roles over periods of time.

What is clear is that there are a number of considerations requiring careful attention when designing, implementing and maintaining peer interventions. It is also refreshing and much needed for these to be highlighted and serve as a bottom-up corrective to the seemingly rose-tinted perspectives on peer support as being the golden panacea for prisoner and prison issues. One of the paramount issues that beset peer intervention in England and Wales is a wholesale lack of robust evidence into the effectiveness of utilising peers and peer interventions. Devilly et al. (2005), in their analysis of peer support interventions, make a number of recommendations regarding evaluation and monitoring of interventions. They describe evaluation as:

> An integral part of implementing an effective peer program [. . .] it establishes whether the program is meeting its aims and objectives, provides quality assurance to enable them to continue in the future, and enables continuous feedback and improvement.

They recommend both evaluations of the process or peer intervention and of the impact that it has to deliver its outcomes. Despite this recommendation, Fletcher and Batty (2012) point to a lack of evidence demonstrating a clear added benefit of utilising peer support, with the interventions existing still being 'new, small scale' (Fletcher & Batty, 2012, p. 15) and largely undervalued. Looking further forward, Woodall et al. (2015) indicated, akin to other research into peer interventions, that they may be effective at improving or maintaining the health and well-being of prison populations, but they go on to call for research to validate these claims. This is due to there being 'major research gaps in understanding the role, effectiveness and value of peer interventions within the criminal justice sector' (Woodall et al., 2015, p. 13). When considering this powerful statement, it is perhaps best to exercise caution and view peer intervention in the vein of Milburn (1995, p. 21) who contends that it is 'no more than a working hypothesis rather than a proven model'. With the significant challenges surrounding power-sharing, managerialism and occupational cultures, confidentiality and risk, it is these areas that are considered in this book. In doing so, it draws upon the empirical study into peer-led induction, to address, in part, the aforementioned void in research and develop what understanding that already exists.

Chapter 4

Researching Lived Experience With Lived Experience

> ...we, as prison researchers, have a moral obligation to keep questioning and investigating prisons and closed and total institutions. It is a scientific duty for prison researchers to contribute to gathering evidence for developing correctional and penal policy within the current penal landscape. (Tubex, 2015)

At this point, I can hear people crying 'Oh no, not another methods chapter'. For some in the academy, we may often hear our students' bemoaning engagement with research methods. It is suggested that 'deans, course directors and lecturers would avoid teaching research methods or having it on their curriculum to avoid dealing with student dissatisfaction and complaints' (Czarnecka & Massaro, 2021). Through an autobiographical lens, as both a student and a lecturer, I identify with the notion that there is somewhat of a weariness towards methods. However, we do live in a world that calls for data to be used as an evidence base, and as such, it is therefore crucial to reflect on the process, and what interacts with it, that produces it.

This chapter should not be viewed as one that alienates an audience through prioritising technical jargon laden language that makes engagement and understanding difficult. That is not to say that there is not a place for such considerations nor do I intend to diminish them in any manner. Rather, it intends to shift away from some of the more traditional considerations to one engaging with real-world applicability to explore the interaction of lived experience with the research process, which has become much more prominent in contemporary criminological research.

The incorporation of lived experience is progressively being acknowledged within and across the criminal justice sector and the field of criminology. Over the past 20 years, people with lived experience of the criminal justice system have played an increasingly recognised and respected role within criminal justice contexts. Many public services and institutions, for example the NHS, mental

Navigating Mental Health in the Male Open Prison, 61–83

Published under exclusive licence by Emerald Publishing Limited
doi:10.1108/978-1-83549-706-720251004

health services or drug treatment programmes, have a heritage of involving and hiring people with lived experience. In terms of criminal justice, this commonly entails individuals drawing on their experiences of being criminalised to: support their peers within the system in a variety of CJS programmes, schemes and projects, take up positions in justice organisations, sit on advisory boards and working groups, collaborate on research projects, inform the design of methodological tools or push forward academic debates (Buck, 2020; CJA, 2019; Schreeche-Powell, 2025; Stevens et al., 2025). The benefits of drawing on lived experience to improve the system for others are starting to be increasingly recognised. As a result, actively engaging individuals with lived experience in the research process is desirable (Antojado & McPhee, 2024), and there has been a pronounced shift towards a more rapid and comprehensive integration into criminology, which had previously demonstrated a cautious approach (Fletcher & Batty, 2012; Perrin, 2017; Schreeche-Powell, 2025; South et al., 2014; Stevens et al., 2025). An increasing focus on the value of lived experience perspectives within criminal justice contexts is a positive development acknowledging the value of another kind of 'knowledge' that actively engages the lived experiences of those formerly imprisoned in research, pedagogy and activism in the criminal justice sector (Earle, 2014, 2018; Richards & Ross, 2001; Schreeche-Powell, 2023, 2025).

The term 'lived experience' has its origins in phenomenology though historically it has been focused on participants as the 'subject' of research rather than as active contributors (Dembele et al., 2024; Frechette et al., 2020). Lived experience researchers are people who carry out research with knowledge and experience gained when they have lived or are living through a phenomenon. According to Gupta et al. (2023, p. 3), 'the lived experience researcher role requires the researcher to draw on their lived experiences in the research they conduct and through which they interpret data'. There is an increasing recognition of the complexity of prison environments and the need for evidence-based approaches to enhance prisoner and staff experience (Miličević et al., 2025). Including the perspectives of individuals with lived experience in prisons in the research process can facilitate the effective transfer of research findings to inform prison policy and practice. Involving those with lived experience in research is an area that while harnessing the potential to yield unique insight also yields its own uniqueness in relation to how that experience interacts with the process of conducting the research. The benefits of mobilising inclusion of people with lived experience as producers of research are encouraging (Dembele et al., 2024; Jewkes, 2012; Lamb et al., 2020; Liebling, 1999).

Researching those who have been imprisoned and prison staff is not an easy endeavour. It is important to recognise that both ex-prisoners and current serving staff can be described as hard-to-reach populations. 'Hard-to-reach' is a term used to describe those sub-groups of the population that are difficult to reach or involve in research (Shaghaghi et al., 2011). Hard-to-reach populations are generally floating populations and socially invisible, thus gaining access to them poses major barriers for their recruitment. Hard-to-reach populations may also actively try to suppress their identity and perspectives due to fear of confrontation with legal authorities or simply because of social pressure they feel from other members of the broader community (Shaghaghi et al., 2011). This is especially relevant when taking into consideration the inmate code (Liebling & Maruna, 2005; Sykes, 1958) and prison officer cultures (Arnold et al., 2007; Crawley & Crawley, 2007; Liebling et al., 2011).

Considering the impact on the researcher themselves, they can be put in emotionally challenging situations and ones connected to intersections of power, ownership, agency and voice (Dickson-Swift et al., 2007; Fenge et al., 2019). Another layer to the complexity arises when the researcher is a former prisoner, having served a sentence of imprisonment across Category B, C and D public prisons in England and Wales and as such adding his own lived experience into the methodological mixer. It has been argued that methodological debates surrounding the positionality of those engaged in prison research, while not absent, has been neglected (Brown & Bos, 2017; Phillips & Earle, 2010). As such, there is the opportunity to further illuminate the notion of 'doing lived experience research, with lived experience' through consideration of this positionality in the research process. The chapter draws out the ways in which my positionality as a former prisoner has interacted with the research process. Merton's 'Insider Doctrine' (1972) is directly applicable to my identity. Earle (2014) identifies that, in a research context, there is a difference between 'serving time' and 'spending time' in prison, with Beyens et al. (2015, p. 74) arguing that 'whatever researchers might do, their experiences cannot be compared between the research subject and the researchers'. I, however, bridge this chasm and fall under the category of an 'Insider' which Merton (1972, p. 21) considers as 'the members of specified groups and collectives or occupants of specified social statuses: Outsiders are non-members'. That said, the chapter also argues that I, like many others, am able to hold multiple statuses and as such do not fit neatly within each boundary; in fact, I transcend across an exclusive categorisation of insider or outsider and, as such, straddle both in a manner that is indicative of the 'dynamic rhythms of multi-positionalities' (Ryan, 2015, p. 2) and also symbolic of the liminality of the research space I occupied. The chapter also considers the impact of this researcher positionality upon the recruitment of the prison officer sample of the study through the use of gatekeepers and considers the concepts of prison officer culture that underpin notions of wariness and weariness towards both myself and the research in light of my positionality.

Given that positionality, a sustained reflective approach in the research process is key as 'personal and social characteristics, feelings or emotions, and behaviour may not only facilitate and illuminate but also restrict and distort data and its analysis' (Hammersley, 2015, p. 25). As such, the chapter concludes with consideration of the how I adopted and applied the reflective framework of Dickson-Swift et al. (2007) to consider my reflections on the research process thematically, from the perspective of one researching those with a shared lived experience, the emotional challenges of researching in these contexts and how the process interacts with this identity.

There is a lot of complexity, as I have established thus far, and navigating this complexity requires a great deal of planning precision. That complexity grows exponentially when you factor in an unexpected global pandemic, and it is key to both recognise and use this as a vehicle to illustrate the fluidity and flux of research in the social world. Given turmoil that society has been plunged into in recent times, due to the global crisis experienced as a result of the COVID-19 pandemic, the chapter firstly considers how it has impacted the research process, presenting the challenges and changes that have been made to conducting the research study, both in midst of this global pandemic with a shift from an ethnographic study in the purest sense to one with 'ethnographic edges' (Davies, 2015). This is the chapter's first foray into how we as researchers must embrace and adapt to change – our social world is fluid and so must we be in research.

Research in a Global Pandemic

Like many researchers worldwide, foreseeing a global pandemic that would plunge society into chaos and uncertainty was not a consideration when conceiving and developing the methodological design of the research study upon which this book is based. Methods of data collection that both became and are susceptible to being adversely impacted by COVID-19 include those that involve human interaction, such as interviews and ethnographic research. Due to these factors, qualitative researchers had to adjust their data collection tools, alter their design frames and examine alternatives. In the face of such challenges, however, we as researchers must adapt, and this involves, as Hennekam (2019, p. 1) sets out, 'adapting our research design to the particularities of the population under study, stressing that it is important to stay flexible and open to change at any stage of the research process'. This is not just time-bound to COVID-19, which is merely an illustrative vehicle; rather, this is extended to the wider contextual and environmental settings that this population under study and the study itself is immersed within and any manner of real-world crises could occur that necessitate this adaptability in our research design. The general essence is that whatever we may face, it is being adaptable and creative that increases the probability of us as researchers garnering the very data that we seek by using different research designs and approaches (Hennekam, 2019).

The Changing Face of the Design Frame

In order to achieve the aims and objectives of the empirical study upon which this book is based, the original data collection was scheduled to take the form of face-to-face semi-structured qualitative interviews within the prison environment. The sample pool was identified across four Category D open prisons situated in England and Wales. The prisoner sample inclusion criteria were scheduled to comprise solely of adult male prisoners received into custody at four identified Category D open prisons in the South of England, following transfer from a 'closed conditions' prison. The prison induction officers' sample had a criterion that stipulated that they be required to have at least 1 year experience in the induction function at their institution and in-depth working knowledge and experience of their role and prisoner facing experience of induction processes and procedure in relation to transfer and induction. The Peer Support Workers (due to the transient nature and frequent turnover associated with the regime of open prisons) were required to be in post as a Peer Support Worker at their institution for a minimum of 3 months. The study sought those willing to talk about their experiences in the role of a Peer Support Worker and its nature as well as their observations of this interaction with mentees and on relations between staff, prisoners and peers.

So far so good, yet there is always a but! As most penal researchers are aware, wanting to conduct research with staff and/or offenders in prison establishments requires formal research approval to the HMPPS National Research Committee (NRC). In response to the threat of COVID-19, the MOJ and HMPPS took action to protect staff and people accommodated in prisons or on supervision in the community. This involved making significant alterations to ways of working and implementing restrictions to limit the movement of people. Based on these restrictions, the NRC introduced a moratorium on primary research in HMPPS. The moratorium aimed to ensure safety and reduce unnecessary burden on the prison and probation estate. As such, all research studies were suspended. Additionally, submitted research applications were not processed, and prospective applications were unable to be submitted. At the time, there was no timeline as to when the HMPPS research application process would re-open nor were there any indications of changes to processes and procedures to ensure research applications would be COVID-19 regulation compliant.

With this in mind, and with the ethnographic fieldwork originally scheduled on an ever-impending timeline, the decision was made to adapt the design frame, both to ensure timeframes were met but also following consideration of both the potential and actual logistical challenges as introduced. The changes were that data collection no longer took place within the prison and took place in community settings, and as such, participant observation was no longer an element of the study. The sample was changed with the intended prisoner sample now becoming an ex-prisoner population. Prison staff involved in the process of induction were still recruited; however, this occurred outside of the prison environment via social media and gatekeeper staff due to the lack of what can be termed as a captive audience. They were also interviewed outside of the prison in community settings. The peer mentee prisoner sample also changed from prisoners currently serving sentences of imprisonment to ex-prisoners released into the community, which removed the need to enter the custodial setting, and they were recruited through NGO and CJS organisations and interviewed in community settings, and finally, Prisoner Peer Support Workers were removed from the sample to reflect that physical access to the custodial setting has now been removed from the study. As such, this group were no longer to be accessed, and the sample size was reduced. It was, however, the abandoning of an ethnographic study in its purest construction that prompted the most significant consideration and change.

'Why Be on the Inside When You Can Do It on the Out?'

Ethnography, as a research methodology, has a rich history that emphasises comprehending the viewpoints of the subjects and monitoring their daily activities (Hammersley & Atkinson, 1983). Ethnographers seek to generate comprehensive and intricate narratives of individuals and the social dynamics in which they are situated. Consequently, it is frequently utilised by researchers in social sciences across diverse institutional, community and other social contexts (Drake et al., 2015). Prison ethnography presents unique challenges as a methodology for investigating prison life.

Some contend that with the life of prisoners, ethnography does not constitute 'genuine' ethnography in the strictest sense of the term, as the predominant body of prison ethnography or prison-related study is conducted by individuals who are unlikely to experience imprisonment themselves. The majority are therefore 'outsiders' who have not directly participated in the experiences those imprisoned and the prison. They do not experience the deprivations of prisoners, and they can hand in their keys at the end of the day and return to their own life outside of the prison walls. The external researcher consistently maintains that option, thereby becoming detached from the reality of the prisoners' experience. As such, immersion is transient rather superficial, especially for ethnographies concentrated on the prisoner society (Drake et al., 2015). Drake et al. (2015, p. 3) define ethnography as 'a form of in-depth study that includes the systematic and impressionistic recording of human cultural and social life in situ. It includes observing and/or interacting with people as they go about their everyday lives, routines and practices'. They contend that purely interview-based research methodologies that tend to be episodic, short-lived and often take place outside of spaces the informant routinely occupies sit in contrast to ethnographic study. Yet as Hammersley (2015, p. 29) rightly observes, the discipline of social science provides 'a wealth of theoretical and empirical resources with which to formulate the context...for the purposes of enquiry....which resources are of use and how they should be interpreted and used must be shaped by our developing understanding of the particular phenomenon we are studying and there questions we are seeking to answer'.

This is precisely what the research study did, in response to the challenges faced. Therefore, the primary method adopted in the empirical study was semi-structured interviews. The interviews took place remotely through mediums such as Zoom and MS Teams. This was born out of limitations regarding face-to-face contact given the COVID-19 pandemic and the associated ethical and institutional demands. So while it is not a traditional ethnographic study in the sense of what we as social scientists often recognize, it still drew on ethnographic methodology and principles in its enactment. It very much aligns with the observations of Davies (2015, p. 467) who conducted research with 'ethnographic edges', as he had shared the experiences that his participants had lived/were living.

Fieldwork entails conducting interviews to uncover knowledge that is otherwise inaccessible; it aims to identify the mental constructs, ideas and values that motivate human behaviour (Holy & Stuchlik, 1983). Understanding the human experience is a fruitless endeavour without listening, as individuals reveal their experiences (Cohen & Rapport, 1995). As Holy and Stuchlik (1983, p. 36) assert, observation alone will not do, and they assert that 'if we do not want simply to observe and report physical movements of people in temporal and spatial sequences, but to study and explain their actions, we can do it only by relating them, implicitly or explicitly, to some notions about such movements to knowledge, beliefs, ideas or ideals'.

The position of Hockey and Forsey (2012, p. 73), is that participant observation may well be the 'most effective way to arrive at the final destination in some, and perhaps even most, cases, but it is not essential to the effective production of a descriptive-analytical account of a social grouping', is one that I embrace strongly. The interviewees in the study were able to show an awareness and highlight their social world in interesting ways. As Hockey and Forsey (2012, p. 76) advance, 'they are quite capable of offering to the interviewer the sorts of insights that are often said to flow most readily from ethnographic/participant observer studies'. The interview is a moment of connection, a site of participation in the world and life of the individual that we spend time with and interact with. It allows us to enter and tap into the knowledge that these individuals have about their experience. That does not mean that we as researchers abandon our ethnographic foundations or principles, but rather, we operationalise the interview with an 'ethnographic imaginary' that commits us to understanding the lived experience of the participant by 'asking about and listening closely to the beliefs, the values, the material conditions and structural forces that underwrite the socially patterned behaviours.... along with the meanings people attach to these conditions and forces' (Forsey, 2010, p. 567). Drawing on the work of Hockey, it is argued that interviews reflect and replicate the realities of social interactions that are often 'spatially dislocated, time-bounded and characterized by intimacy at a distance' (Hockey, 2002, p. 211). This ultimate reinforces that we do not have to observe them to know about them, and as Hockey and Forsey (2012, p. 84) articulate, 'people are very capable of "showing" us at least some of the intricacies of their lives through what they tell us through projects of engaged listening'. Interviews therefore allow us to get 'inside people's heads' for a while.

Given the unprecedented nature of the COVID-19 pandemic, the challenge to create a viable sample and reconstruct the study was a taxing one that required a lot of time and resource intense focus to achieve. The design frame has had some significant changes with the revised parameters of the study, especially surrounding recruitment of the sample and the sampling strategy employed. As there was now no longer what could be described as access to a captive sample pool to recruit form within the prison, the methodology to recruit evolved. There were a number of media and sampling strategies employed as such in order to gain the required sample. Even after reaching and recruiting individuals from a such a population, there existed at times some anxiety stemming from the perceived threat from the authorities among those officers currently serving, when doing research. There was also a hyper-sensitivity surrounding agreeing to cooperate in the study and potential violation of anonymity among the officer sample.

In relation to the ex-prisoner sample, the sample was recruited still adopting a purposive approach, and while the prisoner officer sample adopted the same approach, it also arguably contained elements of convenience and snowballing in relation to its composition, as it was recruited through a gatekeeper. This involved identifying and selecting individuals or groups of individuals that are especially knowledgeable about or experienced with a phenomenon of interest (Palinkas et al., 2015), which in this case was prison induction. In this case, the key criteria of the ex-prisoner sample were experience of transfer to open prison and experience of being a mentee within a peer induction programme while for the officer sample, it was experience of facilitating and delivering peer-led induction in an open prison. Recruitment of the ex-prisoner sample took place largely through advertisements on social media platforms, such as Twitter and Facebook, and through targeted emails to members of prison reform organisations. It also drew upon the identification of ex-prisoners through the informal networks that I had assembled throughout my time imprisoned and post-release.

Given the relative paucity of research and theory relating to the experience of open imprisonment and the experience of power applications in that custodial environment and a lack of specificity from what does exist, this served as a rationale for carrying out a grounded theory analysis, since there is limited ability to theorise about this phenomenon. Described as 'the most widely employed interpretive strategy in the social sciences today' (Lincoln & Denzin, 1994, p. 204), grounded theory (Glaser & Strauss, 1967) is the analytical approach and methodology employed in the analysis of this study. The core tenet of grounded theory is to generate and develop theory inductively from data, and as such, if theory is generated from data, the theory will be grounded in data. For the purpose of this study, this approach to analysis drew upon the 'systematic approach to analysis' model, allowing a more detailed process in relation to the classification, sorting and arrangement of information to examine the relationships in the data. A number of themes and subsequent conceptualisations emerged throughout the study and were integrated into the research as it developed. The culmination of the phases is represented in the thematic findings.

There are inevitably debates surrounding sample sizes in qualitative research and the strengths and limitations of using a 'small sample'. However, in using a small sample, this study can disseminate an in-depth insight into the experiences of adult males experiencing transition, transfer and the induction intervention as well as of those staff members in the delivery and facilitation of the intervention. It does not claim to be representative of all individuals within the criminal justice system experiencing and involved in these processes. Martel (2004, p. 170) suggests that such 'small samples and generate (in)valuable insights about the particular, or "local", character of our global world'. In this vein, while not data that are representative of all prisoners or all staff, what it does allow for is a detailed, visceral portrayal of a smaller number. As such, in my fieldwork for the study, I embraced the concept of Wolcott's (1990, p. 63) 'do less, more thoroughly' as its motto.

Positionality

Research 'represents a shared space, shaped by both the researcher and participants' (England, 1994); therefore, it is always key to remember that the identities of these actors have the potential to impact the research process. In drawing upon the work of Gadamer (2013) and Savolainen et al. (2023, p. 2) advance that 'each person has a historically and culturally situated position, the locus of a horizon – a standpoint that simultaneously enables and limits one's vision'. Positionality has emanated from 'feminist, post-structuralist and postcolonial traditions that have sought to challenge the methodological hegemony of neopositivist empiricism' (England, 1994; Sanghera & Thapar-Bjorkert, 2008). The feminist iteration of knowledge situation comprises three of relevance to fieldwork: situated knowledge which is simply what we can know is shaped by our experiences and social location, epistemic privilege where those with lived experience are presumed to be better positioned to access truths about the social world and achievement whereby there is active engagement to illuminate otherwise invisible truths (Savolainen et al., 2023). As such, positionality frames these relationships in the field and acts as a form of governance of the tone of research (Sanghera & Thapar-Bjorkert, 2008).

When undertaking fieldwork, it must be acknowledged that 'research is a process, not just a product' (England, 1994, p. 82). It is said that positionality in research 'reflects the position that the researcher has chosen to adopt within a given research study' (Savin-Baden & Major, 2013, p. 71) and identified by locating the researcher to the concepts of the subject, the participants and the research process and contents. The multidimensional notions of the self-relating to privilege and aspects of social identity – such as identification with a protected characteristic relating to race, nationality, gender and sexual orientation among others – influence researcher positionality. This is further extended to lived experience and the sharing of experiences among a cohort of peers. In this study, the most pertinent aspect of positionality is the notion of personal experience which falls within the category of subjective and contextual positionality (Chiseri-Strater, 1996).

For myself as the researcher to carry out the research methodologies and analysis clearly and accurately as well as construct, critique and articulate my positionality, a reflexive approach is required. Cohen et al. (2011, p. 225) have emphasised that 'researchers should acknowledge and disclose their own selves in the research, seeking to understand their part in it or influence on the research'. In what follows, I consider how my positionality as a former prisoner who served a long-term determinate sentence of imprisonment totalling 15 years in the England and Wales prison estate interacts with the research process, its design, outputs and interpretations.

Insider, Outsider or Somewhere in Between?

> In order to explain a cultural product, it is necessary to know it. And to know it, in matters of thought and emotion, is to have experienced it. (Bronislaw Malinowski, anthropologist, 1884–1942)

When considering the changes in the social world, there is a frequent problematisation around the notion of differentials among and across social groups in relation to accessing diverse types of knowledge. As Merton (1972, p. 11) muses, certain groups have monopolistic accesses to particular kinds of knowledge while others have 'privileged accesses with other groups able to acquire that knowledge but with an elevated level of risk and cost in doing so'. As such, this is conceptualised through the 'Insider and Outsider' doctrines.

In relation to being an Insider, there is the presentation of a new credentialism as 'one of ascribed status, in which understanding becomes accessible onto to the fortunate few or many who are to the manner born' (Merton, 1972, p. 14). Insiders are defined as 'members of specified groups and collectives or occupants of specified statuses; Outsiders are non-members' (Merton, 1972, p. 21). These conceptualisations serve to distinguish between insider access to knowledge and outsider exclusion from it and the ability to understand the group. It is postulated that the authentic understanding of group life can be achieved only by those who are directly embedded within it. As a former prisoner, having served a sentence in public prisons in England and Wales, I can firmly be identified as an 'Insider' among who could be described as my 'criminal peers'. In that sense we are a cohort who have shared in various guises the lived experiences of imprisonment and the day-to-day pain associated with the existence within the walls and institution.

However, as Merton (1972, p. 22) correctly professes, 'we are all, both Insiders and Outsiders'. A Mertonian position is that an individual does not simply hold a single status, they have 'a complement of variously interrelated statuses, which interact to affect both their behaviour and perspective' (Merton, 1972, p. 22). The key term here is complement. These statuses do not have to been constructed or perceived as adversarial, demarcated into an 'us vs them' dichotomy. As Merton rightly exerts, the occupations of these varying statuses, which have differing levels of attributed importance to us as individuals and differing situations and social contexts, activate the differing statuses which then take in that instance precedence and become salient over the other statuses. Therefore, the boundaries between statuses and the Insider and Outsider are permeable and fluid rather than fixed, and while situations arise, different statuses become activated and the lines of separation shift (Merton, 1972).

Being perceived as an Outsider at times has benefits. As Simmel (1950) frequently stated, 'one need not to be Caesar in order to understand Caesar'. Resonating with Simmel's ideas, who postulated that the Outsider is not bound by commitments of allegiance to the group, I felt freer, practically and theoretically, and, as such, was able to seamlessly become more objective in my inquiry. Being an outsider or being perceived as an outsider by those interviewed for the study, rather than being seen as a negative issue acting as a barrier to the richness and depth of data, was instead harnessed positively and, as Simmel (1950, pp. 404–405) muses, allowed me to 'survey with less prejudice [. . .] more objective ideals [. . .] not tied down in my action by habit, piety, and precedent'. It is the very nature of being an Outsider in this framing that allowed me to question things more intently and with greater depth due to adopting at times unfamiliarity. This unfamiliarity was present certainly when engaging with the prison officer sample and also when dealing with some demographics and experiences of imprisonment, especially surrounding those serving indeterminate sentences who viewed me as an Outsider in terms of being able to understand the experience of their sentence despite viewing me as one of their number in relation to being someone who has experienced imprisonment.

Here the fragility of status and the multiplicity or statuses that we hold simultaneously is exposed. As Merton (1972, p. 44) rightly states, 'Insiders and Outsider in the domain of knowledge, unite. You have nothing to lose but your claims. You have a world of understanding to win'. The interchange between these often adversarial viewed and exclusive concepts saw me adopting perspectives to achieve the research aims through my willingness and ability to straddle the multiple statuses and positions of Insider and Outsider, occupying a more dynamic role dependent on the context and situation and guided by the search for rich data form those participants I encountered. As such, positionalities are fluid and adaptable dependent on the interaction in research, and no one identity should be emphasised to the point where other personalities are excluded from the research endeavour (McGarry, 2016).

There are, however, tensions between Insider and Outsider statuses, and the research context was indicative of the idea that I was occupying a performative liminal space whereby I moved 'in and out' not just of my participants' experiences but also my own lived experience. In this construct, I no longer belonged to my old world or to my new one, and I was temporarily in a no man's land (Moran, 2013; Van Gennep, 1909). This also led to confusion because in terms of my identity, I had, in my mind, followed the three stages of passage, separating from my previous life, transitioned and then established myself into a new life. Yet here I was, through conducting research with ex-prisoners and prison staff and their experiences, being dragged back towards my previous identity (Schreeche-Powell, 2019). I was experiencing the liminal experience repeatedly, being in a suspended state betweenness in terms of insider and outsider roles and identity during the research process, from which it was difficult to emerge. However, what the engagement with the liminal phases, places and states afforded me was the opportunity to consider the experience of navigating my transition in differing contexts through a newly defined lens to question my sense of self (Cook-Sather, 2006; Ibarra & Obodaru, 2016). I was engaging in a constant process of 'Identity Work' where I was forming, repairing, maintaining strengthening and revising my identity, as I was adapting within the boundaries of a previous identity, yet seeking to maintain authenticity while also adapting to my new identity as a researcher. What is apparent is that 'researching lived experience, with led experience', leads to betwixt and between experiences that must be recognised and navigated when conducting research.

Merton (1972, p. 19) argues that groups 'want to make their interpretation the prevailing one of how things were and are and will be', and it is important that this research therefore captures what Heidegger (1976) terms a public interpretation of reality. Merton (1972) suggests that 'the critical measure of success is when the interpretation moves beyond the boundaries of the ingroup to be accepted by the Outsider', and as such, I adopt this critical measure of success when assessing the relevance and success of the dissemination of both the narrative findings in this book but also the insights I can convey to those who engage with this book in whatever guise. Moreover, it is an interpretation that is applied in practice to improve the experience of imprisonment for those who are imprisoned. As for my identity, the outcome of this study may well also activate differing statuses in the status set, just as it did in the research process, influencing how I am 'claimed' as an Insider, Outsider or someone in between.

From Gatekeepers to Caretakers: Engaging With the Prison Officer

With the changes to the study, accessing a prison officer sample became challenging. While my insider status was able to facilitate the effective recruitment of the ex-prisoner sample, it was a more complex process for officers, especially given the research existed independently of the NRC framework. I attempted through social media to recruit officers for the study, yet this yielded no responses whatsoever. As such, I relied on a senior operational HMPPS officer as a gatekeeper to provide access to a sample of prison officers willing to engage with both myself and the research. It is a complex, ongoing process that has a powerful impact on the extent to which a research study is successful. Gatekeepers are defined as 'those individuals in an organization that have the power to withhold (or allow) access to people or situations for the purposes of research' (De Laine, 2000, p. 123) It is acknowledged that those gatekeepers play a pivotal role in social research, particularly when researching communities that do not trust mainstream research and are seldom heard or for research involving sensitive subjects (Eide & Allen, 2005). To access participation sensitively and meaningfully from groups for research, researchers have identified gatekeepers as important mediators, an approach I adopted to ensure the most appropriate sample of participants are both identified and recruited.

The role of the gatekeeper is often influenced by a variety of potential factors. Motivation remains a crucial factor. Intrinsic motivation is a powerful tool in stimulating individuals to engage especially if there is a sense of achievement, personal satisfaction and ownership in the process. Extrinsic factors relate to a supportive working environment for research. Both forms of motivation were at play and observed during the study, and it was evident that the combination of being involved in the research process, a clear understanding of the rationale behind the research and its need in gaining recognition from the researcher all contributed to positive attitudes and behaviours (McFadyen & Rankin, 2016). This gatekeeper I negotiated with for access was known to me through a mutual activity outside of the prison environment and had gotten to know me over a period of time. This individual was supportive in their manner, engaging in their ideas and thoughtful in conversations. It became apparent to me that this individual was concerned with the operationalisation and managerialism of the current prison system and that officers were being diverted away from developing relationships with prisoners and supporting them.

While this was a refreshing perspective, I harboured initial concerns that the sample generated by the gatekeeper could be skewed by virtue of the gatekeeper selecting a sample that shared their perspective of prison management and how it was operationalised. A key notion to mitigate this was acceptance that it was not a representative sample, but I have the belief that people who give up their time to be interviewed do so because they share values for increasing understanding of a social phenomenon. It is almost akin to a sense of their responsibility and duty to respect the value of research and their own privilege to be able to shape change. I put trust in the gatekeeper's apparent genuine passion for positive change and interest in how my work fitted within such a continuum, alongside a level of pre-existing trust, rapport and reciprocity between the gatekeeper and myself. Given my positionality as an ex-prisoner, the gatekeeper was important as they recruited access to those officers who they deemed to be willing to be involved and who would also offer value to the cause of the research. The gatekeeper also acted almost as a guarantor of the researcher's legitimacy and that of the research too (De Laine, 2000). My faith regarding a suitable sample being selected was qualified once the sample had been interviewed, and it was clear that they were a diverse set but all willing to offer insight without a dominant discourse to target management blindly. This resonated with the idea expressed by Hockey and Forsey (2012, p. 73) that 'most who participate in social research interviews take and indeed welcome the opportunity to reveal the processes that constitute an authentic interior self as best they can'.

Of interest was how the gatekeeper positioned me as the researcher, and in this vein, they often related to me first as a friend/associate and as a researcher secondarily. Arguably, 'researchers remain dependent on the goodwill of gatekeepers to a very large extent' (Heath et al., 2004, p. 26), and I was no different. It was the gatekeeper who mediated access and arranged the interviews with the officers whom they provided access to, and I was forewarned 'not to let me [them] down' (Gatekeeper Officer). This was important as there was a natural level of research 'weariness' and 'wariness' (Sanghera & Thapar-Bjorkert, 2008) among a climate of fear and suspicion. I did not want to let down the gatekeeper, especially as I was all too aware of the potential recrimination that I could face in the context of my research from the gatekeeper who had the power to limit the conditions for access to participants and limiting access to respondents.

This was illustrated in both the furtive and sensitive nature that communications with the gatekeeper took place. The gatekeeper made it clear that communications should not take place via email or phone, nor should text messages be used, only a brief WhatsApp message (an encrypted medium and as such untraceable) requesting to catch up could be used and that the gatekeeper would make the contact and would primarily meet in person to discuss anything that needed attention relating to the research process. The gatekeeper explained that they were naturally suspicious and risk-averse as after all it was their job to be like that. I was sympathetic and understanding to this and supported those interactions and communications to exist free from the shackles of hyper-vigilance and suspicion.

One of the key questions frequently asked by prison officer participants recruited by the gatekeeper related to who I was, why I was doing this study and why people should communicate with me about their experiences of their role and day to day job. Minority or marginalised communities are often misrepresented, pathologised or problematised by research processes, and prison officers have often had a maligned identity and viewed in some realms as inferior and as deficit. Prison has been established so far as a medium for pain delivery, dehumanising for those experiencing it, and this includes staff. So despite some initial bristling by myself in response towards challenges of my motivations and integrity, I remained mindful in my interactions with officers of Scott's (2006) work. This highlighted prison officers as spending more time in prison than any other occupational group and often longer than those who are imprisoned, and they, too, are subject to pains of imprisonment, whether that be fear, mental health issues, isolation, uncertainty, anxiety and even powerlessness (Crawley, 2005). So, in facilitating and enacting the delivery of pain, they too suffer pain, and they too are dehumanised. Returning to the theorising of Merton (1972), it can be argued that the prison officers provided both Insider and Outsider perspectives, sharing perceptions and understanding in both realms. Therefore, I remained focused on the ideas that the special perspectives and insights that arose from this much-maligned group of staff 'systematically frustrated by the social system: the disinherited, deprived, disenfranchised, dominated and exploited Outsiders' is invaluable to both myself and furthering the field (Merton, 1972, p. 29).

Reflections on the Research

> Viewing one's involvement as both problematic and valid and of recording the subjective experiences of doing research [...] underpin the creation of knowledge. (Gelsthorpe & Morris, 1990, p. 88)

It is accepted that there are dangers associated with a researcher self being made visible in social research (Rowe, 2015). Reflexivity is a proactive process involving the researcher being aware of their effect on the research process, relationships and outcomes of the research. It involves researchers actively acknowledging the implications for the knowledge of the social world they generate, of their methods, values, biases, decisions and where they are positioned and situated in the research itself. It is crucial to have awareness that the underlying prejudices and assumptions we display as social actors can transcend and influence how we can impede rather than facilitate the research process (Enosh & Ben-Ari, 2015; Mead, 1934). After all, 'good qualitative design seeks to understand the self in research' (Lazard & McAvoy, 2020, p. 162). As such, a constant process of reflection is an analysis of the research process on many levels to improving current and future research. It has been defined as being an active process which should result in learning, changing behaviours and practices with processes of reflexive analysis and reflection should be an integrated component of the research study from the beginning (McFadyen & Rankin, 2016). This is an approach that this study embraces.

> Those individuals involved in our research are subjects not objects [. . .] they should not be treated as a chemist would treat a chemical substance or a geologist would treat a rock, The objects of criminological inquiry are not inanimate. (Jupp, 1989, p. 130)

Undertaking prison research requires significant amounts of practical and emotional commitment. By entering the prison world, researchers are able to see a world that few others gain access to, listen to stories that are rarely heard and ask questions that many are interested in (Drake et al., 2015; Garrihy & Walters, 2015; Jewkes, 2012; Liebling, 1999). There is another dimension experience of prison research that is often left under-explored: the emotional challenges and costs that invariably accompany any research into the penal experience. When undertaking the form of research involving human interaction, you will be confronted with the emotionality of them as well as subjects being research. Entering 'the prison world' physically, when conducting research into the prison, is just one aspect of researching the prison world. It is my position that anyone engaging in qualitative enquiry invariably enters the prison world and experiences those emotional challenges, especially amplified when you have a shared experience of that world with your participants. Engaging with this emotion is an area that allows offers the opportunity to become an 'actively engaged emotional researcher' as obfuscating the researcher is akin to severing a link in the chain (Garrihy & Watters, 2020, p. 3). As such, it is important to advance accounts of this engagement, something that has been called for by penal scholars (Jewkes, 2012; Liebling, 1999).

Reflexivity is not just an endeavour putting the researcher at the centre and promoting effective and robust research through improvement. There is a human aspect, and the participants of research must always be a vital component of the reflective process to respect the key tenets of ethical consideration as well as to ensure participant voice is heard. As someone formerly imprisoned, my biographical history provides a lived familiarity with the research participants, all of whom have been subject to imprisonment whether that be as prisoners or as caretakers of punishment (Scott, 2006). However, I do not attempt to speak for the research participants who have a prisoner identity nor do I work on their behalf to challenge any experienced injustice. Rather, I tread carefully in balancing objectivism and subjectivism. There is a range of generic benefits stemming from my 'insider' status when researching from which I have benefitted. Of particular importance was the ease of access to the research participants who are typically acknowledged as a hard-to-reach group by virtue of being considered as 'one of us' (Sanghera & Thapar-Bjokert, 2008, p. 556). I was also able to construct and operationalise more meaningful, probing and insightful questions, together with an ability to understand the offender identity vernacular and language, including body language. In their exploration of conducting sensitive research, Dickson-Swift et al. (2007, p. 330) recognise that when conducting sensitive research, we as researchers are 'going into other people's lives, sometimes at times of crisis and stress, and we ask them to talk in detail about their experiences'. Although it can be painful and revealing for researchers to explore the emotional aspects of their work, the examination of emotions' function has been insufficiently investigated in prison studies despite its significance to the research process (Garrihy & Watters, 2020; Yuen, 2011).

I have already highlighted some manifestations of my positionality which were also considerations when constructing the design frame, and I have adopted a reflective framework of five of the entangled and mutually impacting themes using the scaffolding of Dickson-Swift et al. (2007) for the purpose of this reflection on the research process in what follows:

Self-Disclosure

The process of establishing and developing trust was key to providing an enabling effect upon participants, and as such, giving them the confidence to share sensitive and personal information and reassuring them that the data provided will not be misused or abused (Baxter Magolda, 2004). Disclosure can vary among researchers, and self-disclosure can serve to enhance rapport and reciprocity, but it can also introduce demanding situations where researchers may become vulnerable and emotionally entangled (Dickson-Swift et al., 2007).

Self-disclosure is advanced by Dickson-Swift et al. (2007, p. 343) as being 'often reported as good research practice with some advocating researchers' self-disclosure'. I recognised in the research that my positionality as an offender means that I can be characterised as an 'Insider' such that, by disclosing this positionality, the relationship between myself and the ex-offender participants was viewed by them as less hierarchical; I was able to create a 'level playing field' (Dickson-Swift et al., 2007, p. 332). This also fed into the development of a good rapport with the research participants, and this was a conscious choice by myself, which I feel benefitted the process. There is a danger of being vulnerable through self-disclosure and considerations of what one should or need to disclose. Invariably when researching with lived experience or engaging in any endeavour where lived experience identity is enacted, we invariably give a piece of ourselves to our audience. For me, it is also just not what should or needs to be shared but rather how much of myself do I give. However, as this took place with participants who share the commonality of the first-hand experience of imprisonment, there was no vulnerability experienced, and it was a positive step in the interview process. I chose to openly disclose information about my identity, thoughts and feelings surrounding the plentiful issues within the penal system in England and Wales, including my own beliefs regarding the impact of peer support interventions, while demonstrating a sympathetic demeanour to participants regarding the realities of day-to-day life as either a prisoner or a prison officer and demonstrating an awareness of the complexities of their roles. This disclosure in particular enabled the gatekeeper and participants to gauge my authenticity and support, overcoming the culture of fear and uncertainty that co-exists with the aforementioned wariness, supporting them in engaging with rich insights.

Despite this, imprisonment is experienced uniquely by each individual subjected to it, and it is a layered effect. Although there was a commonality in the fact I had been imprisoned, the composition of that differed between myself and my peers, especially those serving indeterminate sentences. Here I was viewed more as an Outsider, and I was able to reflect that in some senses I was while also straddling the notion of an Insider on a lesser level. As a researcher and ex-prisoner who served a determinate sentence, my lived experience did not encompass indeterminacy and the extremely specific set of pains and frustrations clearly felt by the participants identifying with that sentence. In fact, a familiar outpouring from those participants was that I would not be able to understand or did not understand what they go through or what it is like to serve that sentence. This served, however, to sharpen my focus and objectivity to explore and garner rich data about an emotive area of prison life that I previously had limited understanding of. As such, it was a learning process for me. The comprehension of an ex-prisoner now researching was viewed with suspicion, especially by those serving indeterminate sentences, and there was a positioning of myself by them at times as aligned with the structures of power meting out the conditions that elicit such powerful and emotive responses of anger and frustration. It was almost to them as if I had crossed over to 'the other side', and as such, there was a strong focus on ensuring that there was constant negotiation in the face of my motivation being tested and tried at times. Suspicion did not stop here when positionality was declared because some wariness from the prison officer sample existed; I was viewed as an Outsider from their cohort and culture, and again, this process of re-enforcing my motivations was key to overcoming this.

Rapport

> It feels weird talking about it [. . .] it seems like a lifetime ago now.
> (Joey)

The most pertinent aspect of qualitative research enquiry, as Dickson-Swift et al. (2007, p. 331) argue, is that 'researchers must initiate a rapport-building process from the first encounter with a participant to build a research relationship that will allow the researcher access to that person's story'. I used my positionality and disclosure of my own experiences of the criminal justice system when interviewing the ex-offender component of the sample frame to facilitate this rapport, which I believe underpinned elevated levels of participant disclosure. I was careful, however, to ensure that the openness and intimacy of the interviews were not leading in any way in the interest of ethics.

> You've been out a while now [. . .] it's changed in that time you've been out; COVID and all that shit changed everything, and we had to live it, you didn't. (Danny)

There was at times some disconnect between me and some of the ex-prisoner sample. Prisons, as well as society post prison, are in constant flux, and as such, this ever-changing context influences the experiences of those exposed to them. Just like I manage a multiplicity of identities, which is often challenging, those that I interviewed also share this. Some are developing existing identities while also creating and developing new identity, all while navigating day to day life, often in a more acute manner than others due to their criminal history and experiences of imprisonment. When you are in prison together as part of the population, there is a greater degree of shared commonality and focus on day-to-day life. The very nature of restriction for those imprisoned means that there are a limited range of opportunities for people. As such, discussions and activity can be limited and akin to 'Groundhog Day'; people doing and talking about the same or similar things, often repetitively. It is easier in this context to interact and demonstrate bonds of commonality. However, freedom has eroded that commonality by virtue of, and exposure to, free will and choice, and this exposes the level of difference between us as individuals.

> I ain't about that anymore [. . .] it will always be a part of me but it's not who I am now or something that I wanna think about too much. (Chris)

It is acutely apparent to me that the shared experience of prison is no longer as dominant as it once was. It undoubtedly interacts with our being, yet, for most, it has retreated into the shadows, not as relevant or just an identity that those interviewed are trying to move away from. This served at times to undermine the ability to build a rapport as I was trying to probe and elicit responses to topics that were not a priority or focal point for some participants or indeed had been buried or compartmentalised by some. The key to unlocking the door was to remain as relaxed and attempt differing tactics. Being consistent and persistent but not pushy as I tried to identify common ground to use as a foundation for inquiry was the approach used that was effective. It was stop-start at times, but once the commonality was identified on some level, it then seemed to cascade into a good narrative flow producing insightful data.

I was surprised by the rapport I managed to build with the prison staff. I was expecting there to be a power imbalance with the staff exerting their authority and power over me, given the prisoner–staff divide and boundaries often enacted in custodial settings which can be adversarial. However, they were extremely open and engaging, sharing stories and vignettes with me openly and being candid about their employee's strengths and weaknesses and the limitations of their work, role and the intervention. Despite staff being guarded in some respects as outlined earlier, and at times viewing my motivations for this research with suspicion, there appeared to be nothing withheld. What resulted was a dialogue that was open in nature. The staff seemed genuinely pleased to be making a positive contribution both to my work and potentially to offender well-being.

Reciprocity

Through self-disclosure, a 'fair exchange' took place, and despite some of the aforementioned challenges, I am of the belief that these principles contributed to the depth and quality of the research process. The reciprocity from disclosing my positionality, and the ability to share vignettes of my first-hand experience of the same conditions and processes that the participants experience certainly lessened the hierarchical nature of the research and gave them something back which I felt was a crucial factor on a personal level, especially as they were 'letting me into their lives', and prevented me in part from falling into the trap of some researchers who either do not afford or deny, agency (Krumer-Nevo & Benjamin, 2010). That is not to say that my identity was illustrative of a complete sameness with the group, yet it did not denote total difference either (Dwyer & Buckle, 2009).

I was in an extremely privileged position, and I wanted to convey to the participants that this was recognised and respected by myself. At the forefront of my mind was the prominent thought that I was privileged to be allowed a private view of another person's past, their pain and their sorrow. Akin to the research of Liamputtong Rice and Ezzy (1999), I was extremely grateful to have this access, and while the research process can be described as laborious at times, I had a renewed vigour and did not feel bogged down by the weight of the work I had undertaken. For me, part of the process of reciprocity was to now harness a responsibility to act upon the information shared and reciprocate further by producing a study that underpins change in the penal establishment.

Feeling Guilty

Reflecting on the research process, I identified that it had left an 'ethical hangover' (Lofland & Lofland, 1995, p. 28), 'the feeling of persistent guilt or unease over what is viewed as a betrayal of the people under study'. I was interviewing my criminal peers, people who share similar first-hand experience of imprisonment and are subjected to the same pains of imprisonment, and they were sharing with me their extremely personal and sensitive experiences, thoughts and emotions, which I was then using with what Etherington (1996, p. 347) would describe as my 'researcher ears' and as a 'means to an ends' (Dickson-Swift et al., 2007, p. 343) in terms of my research aims and objectives. My emotions were spiked by conditions often mirroring those experienced by Liebling (2014, p. 481):

> ...when faced with the challenge of being with and getting to know young, Black, mixed race or White, physically healthy men in their twenties or early thirties who had been sentenced to indeterminate or life sentences with tariffs often longer than their ages. Their condition was simply unmanageable, for them, and for us as their witnesses.

This made me feel uncomfortable and voyeuristic even, indicative of what Dwyer and Buckle (2009) term 'role conflict', that I was 'out' and they were still metaphorically 'in' and living their sentence, albeit in the community, and that I was also exploiting them. In a way, I was and at times reflected on 'loyalty tugs' that arose from my emotions (Dwyer & Buckle, 2009; Glesne & Peshkin, 1992). I was all too aware of 'most research about marginalised people being done by those who are not marginalised' (Buck et al., 2023) and that the impact of this can manifest is experiences being weaponised and distorted leaving minimal footprint in terms of positive impact on the lives of those criminalised and the structural condition that they face.

England (1994, p. 85) is emphatic about this proposition when stating 'exploitation and possibly betrayal are endemic to fieldwork' and some go as far as labelling this the 'violence of fieldwork' (Crapanzano, 1977). While I am mindful of this and the proposition that 'fieldwork might actually expose the researched to greater risk and be more intrusive and more exploitative than more traditional methods' (England, 1994, p. 85), this is not something that was apparent or implicit during the research, and I feel that this was also mitigated by the robust ethical framework put in place. I also felt that this is done in the quest of making things better for those who were now where we had been. I harnessed these emotions to feel a sense of duty to ensure that the research I conducted contributes to making the custodial environment better and improve offender outcomes for my peers currently in custody and entering custody in the future and indeed the people who I interviewed should they return to custody at a later date.

Process of Interview

It is postulated by Ely et al. (1991, p. 49) that 'if we undertake to study human lives, we have to be ready to face human feelings'. With this in mind, and given my own experiences imprisonment, I was comfortable enough not to be affected by considerations of vulnerability or marginalisation as I was among my peers and therefore felt it was appropriate to display 'caring behaviours' – such as compassion, comfort, concern, empathy, compassion interest, sharing and support (Leininger, 1981, p. 13). While most of the sample participants were genial, warm, friendly, curious and keen to be involved and help, what I perhaps was not prepared for was the level of emotion behind the words shared with me. There was anger, rage, frustration, helplessness, resignation across both the ex-prisoner and staff sample that was powerful and delivered in a no-holds barred manner; those individuals did not hold back or measure their delivery. This was exponentially acute among those who served indeterminate sentences.

> No one did fuck all for me when I was in; just left me there to rot in that shithole. (Graeme)

Annison and Condry (2018, p. 2) highlight that:

> . . .a pervasive sense of injustice and uncertainty underpins and permeates more specific concerns relating to efforts to progress towards release and managing the stresses of life beyond release [. . .] Family relationships – both with the prisoner and more widely – are often heavily disrupted [. . .] significant negative health effects caused by the stress and anxiety. All of this is likely to undermine efforts to rehabilitate individuals who have served an Indeterminate sentence.

This indicates a degree of liminality that these individuals both face and navigate on a daily basis. The majority of those participants subject to indeterminate sentences were frequently disengaged from the focus of the questions and engaged instead with a vitriolic critique of the prison system and how it had as one individual described as 'shat on [them] from a great height, every single fucking day' (Joey).

I felt that for these individuals. The engagement for them was cathartic and gave them a voice to be heard, empowering them to have their say as human beings after being subjected to dehumanising environment primarily and secondarily to contribute to change. Aresti et al. (2016) highlight that the 'voices of marginalised groups are effectively and systematically muted and silenced, both in academic research and in the work of statutory and non-statutory organizations in the criminal justice field'. I could have been more focused in my interviewing and steered these men back to the questions at hand however, with the notions of Aresti et al. (2016) ringing in my ears I decided early on to let those men speak their truth and say what they needed to say. After all, what cost was it to me to dedicate some extra of my time to them? The answer was little. As someone formerly imprisoned, I knew extremely well the importance of someone giving you a bit of their time, sometimes just to chat socially and sometimes to allow you to vent your frustrations, whether that be about the system, its treatment of them or a wide range of other personal issues. Theirs are voices which have been silenced or gone unheard for too long and I wanted to ensure that they were heard authentically and given the platform and freedom to do so. Secondary yet and of importance to the research study at hand was the notion that:

> . . .the prisoner's voice is an essential one for exposing bad practice, helping to set standards of decency and acceptability within prison walls and for countering the de-humanization, depersonalization and stigmatization of both prisoners and their families [. . .] To facilitate lasting and effective penal reform and change they demand to be authentically heard. (Aresti et al., 2016, p. 13)

Both elements were impossible to disentangle so I embraced them instead. By being 'methodologically alert' through my positionality and reflexive framework, I was aware of the ways I could have misinterpreted or skewed the experiences shared because of my own experiences. There was, as far is possible, no apparent blurring of boundaries between myself and my participants, and I believe that, by employing these behaviours, I gained a richer and greater depth of insight into the experiences of the participants. I did not present as being unconsciously biased or overly sympathetic to the participant culture and background nor as being too close to the culture. As a result, there was no presence of a myopic view precluding my ability to ask requisite questions to achieve the research aims and objectives nor an inability to introduce and acknowledge an external perspective to the research process. Also, due to the participant knowledge of my Insider status, there was a concern that participants may assume that I possessed a certain amount of expertise or indeed more than I do and that I share a similar understanding, and as such information that may be deemed as obvious to myself may not be disclosed or explained although this did not appear to be the case and rather that I was able to 'tune in' to the differing elements of the experiences shared (Walkerdine et al., 2012, p. 97).

Navigating the Complexity of Lived Experience Research

This chapter has explored the methodological journey of conducting research with lived experience as both a lens and a position. By reflecting on my dual role as both researcher and former prisoner, I have sought to illuminate the ways in which personal history interacts with the research process – not as a limitation but as a source of insight. The chapter has engaged with the complexities of insider/outsider positionality, the ethical and emotional dimensions of researching imprisonment, and the necessity of methodological adaptability in response to real-world challenges – most notably, the COVID-19 pandemic.

One of the key takeaways from this discussion is that positionality is neither fixed nor binary. Rather than being neatly categorised as an 'insider' or 'outsider', I have found myself occupying a liminal space, shifting between roles depending on the context and the nature of my interactions with participants. This fluidity underscores the need for researchers, particularly those with lived experience, to remain reflexive about how their own backgrounds shape the research encounter. At times, my shared history with formerly incarcerated participants created a sense of rapport and trust while in other moments – especially when engaging with prison officers or those serving indeterminate sentences – my position was met with scepticism or wariness. This reinforces the idea that researcher identity is not just about self-perception but is also shaped by how participants interpret and respond to the researcher's presence.

Beyond positionality, this chapter has also highlighted the ethical and emotional responsibilities inherent in conducting research with marginalised or criminalised populations. The process of eliciting deeply personal narratives – often filled with pain, frustration, and trauma – requires more than methodological rigour; it requires a sense of responsibility towards those who share their experiences. The concept of reciprocity in research goes beyond simply extracting data; it involves ensuring that participants feel heard and that their contributions have the potential to inform meaningful change. In this sense, lived experience research is not just about representation but it is about responsibility, ethics and the challenge of honouring participants' voices without appropriating or distorting their experiences.

The necessity of adaptability has also been a central theme in this chapter. The research process was significantly altered by the onset of COVID-19, forcing shifts in methodology, access and participant recruitment. While the initial study design aimed for immersive ethnography within the prison system, the realities of the pandemic necessitated a transition to remote qualitative interviews, a shift that aligned more closely with what Davies (2015) refers to as research with 'ethnographic edges'. Rowe (2015, p. 367) asserts thoughtfully that ethnography 'relies on the perception of the researcher, whose to know the field bodily, intuitively and emotionally, as well as intellectually and through the accounts of others'. While I did not engage with a traditional ethnography, I was still able to harness all of these principles that are shared, and through the injection of my own lived experience and positionality, I was able to substitute 'physical engagement with the field' in a bodily, intuitive and emotional sense. These changes illustrate the importance of flexibility in social research, particularly in criminology, where access to institutions and participants is often constrained by bureaucratic, logistical or political barriers. The ability to pivot – whether due to a global crisis or institutional resistance – is crucial for ensuring that research remains viable and impactful.

Ultimately, this chapter argues that researching lived experience *with* lived experience is a deeply relational and dynamic act. It requires a careful balance between critical distance and empathetic engagement, between recognising one's own biases and ensuring that participant narratives are not filtered through a purely personal lens. The methodological reflections presented here contribute to broader discussions about the role of lived experience researchers in criminology, emphasising that their insights are not only valid but vital to shaping a more nuanced and person-centred understanding of the experience of the penal world.

As the following chapters shift from methodology to their fruits, they build upon this reflexive foundation to explore the experiences of peer-led induction in open prisons. While this chapter has focused on the *process* of research – its challenges, adaptations and theoretical underpinnings – the next sections will consider the *outcomes*, providing deeper insights into the lived experiences of those navigating the prison system.

Chapter 5

Cultures of Knowledge: Structural and Institutional Constraint and Impediment in Peer Support

> Tick box exercise [. . .] a special kind of vacuity that is damaging because the tick does not refer to the reality on the ground. (Boyle, 2021, p. 30)

This chapter explores the impact of peer-led induction on the mental health and well-being of prisoners in open prisons. It examines how this process unfolds during the early transitional days of custody following transfer, a period often marked by entry shock and fear of the unknown. Open prisons are intended to offer a less restrictive penal environment, yet for many prisoners, the transition brings significant psychological distress, uncertainty and adaptation struggles. The knowledge imparted during induction is essential in helping prisoners navigate this unfamiliar environment and early imprisonment. While peer-led induction is positioned as a crucial intervention at a time of potential crisis, this chapter uncovers systemic failures, including a culture of disinterest, self-interest and constraint among both staff and mentors, which ultimately undermine its effectiveness.

The chapter situates peer-led induction within knowledge management and knowledge sharing frameworks, exploring how knowledge is transferred, controlled and restricted within the prison system. Knowledge is power in institutional settings, and in prisons, the flow of knowledge is heavily regulated and constrained by hierarchical structures. Support Workers, despite their role in aiding adaptation, often withhold information, strategically frame knowledge or filter what is shared, reflecting their own experiences of power and control. Similarly, prison officers and management often engage in a bureaucratic, tick-box approach, reducing induction to a mechanical process rather than a meaningful intervention.

Navigating Mental Health in the Male Open Prison, 85–109

Published under exclusive licence by Emerald Publishing Limited
doi:10.1108/978-1-83549-706-720251005

Gupta et al. (2000, p. 19) highlight that successful knowledge sharing requires organisations to 'convince, coerce, direct or otherwise get people' to share information. In an environment where trust is low and self-preservation dominates, the effectiveness of peer-led induction becomes compromised. This is particularly problematic in the early days of arrival. The emotional weight of entry shock and adaptation stress is profound, as prisoners grapple with the reality of their new conditions, uncertain expectations and the challenge of adjusting to a prison culture that is simultaneously restrictive yet unfamiliar in its freedoms.

Building on Sykes' (1958) and Crewe's (2011a, 2011b) theories on the pains of imprisonment, this chapter extends these frameworks by considering the unique pains of transfer and adaptation in open prisons. Unlike in closed conditions, where confinement and security dictate experience, open prisons introduce new anxieties, unpredictability and self-regulation, which can be conceptualised a contributing to 'double liminality'. Here transitioning from their former world (the closed prison) to their present world (the open prison) while simultaneously preparing for re-entry to their future world can be understood through this framework. This transition involves navigating the uncertainties of a less restrictive prison environment and the impending challenges of societal re-entry, each with its own set of expectations and uncertainties. The pain of transfer, transition and adaptation is not merely logistical but deeply psychological, as prisoners experience the destabilising effects of moving from a rigidly controlled system to one that places more responsibility on them.

This chapter also critically examines the formal expectations of prison induction. While policies suggest that new prisoners should be supported, the reality of the experience is shaped by managerialism, tokenistic implementation and a disengaged workforce. The gap between policy and practice creates additional distress for prisoners, as induction becomes more about bureaucratic compliance than meaningful support. The findings suggest that both mentors and staff contribute to this culture of inefficiency and disinterest. Many prisoners report that induction is reduced to a 'tick-box, bean-counting culture' that prevents prison officers from connecting with offenders (The Guardian, 2013). Instead of fostering a supportive and needs-driven environment, induction is carried out as a bureaucratic obligation, lacking genuine engagement with the struggles of prisoners adjusting to open conditions. Finally, the chapter explores structural barriers to effective peer-led induction, including ineffective leadership, staff resistance and competing institutional interests. Prison officers often viewed peer-led induction as a challenge to their authority. The shift towards power-sharing between staff and prisoners unsettles traditional penal identities, reinforcing a culture of disengagement, distrust and resistance to change.

Despite these challenges, there are pockets of good practice where peer-led induction demonstrates potential. However, for it to be truly effective needs driven model in improving mental health and adaptation outcomes, the systemic barriers must first be addressed.

The Foundations of Knowledge Management and Knowledge Sharing

> Knowledge is lifeblood of an organization, and it has been identified as a crucial element for the survival of organizations. It implies that managing knowledge is as important for an organization as other assets are managed. In order to be successful, organizations heavily depend on knowledge that has become a resource and critical success factor. (Asrar-ul-Haq & Anwar, 2016, p. 1)

Knowledge sharing operates in institutional environments characterised by uncertainty, change and instability that lead to the creation of various challenges. Issues emerge from these factors which require organisations to quickly and easily adapt to them. The prison is no different. The documented issues surrounding mental health and safer custody of those imprisoned has led to the prison responding by introducing interventions and measures to bring about positive outcomes. The success of such organisational measures is highly dependent on knowledge sharing and knowledge management (Fong et al., 2011). Insights, interpretations, context, experience and wisdom are all examples of knowledge, and they all help an organisation achieve its objectives, mission and vision while also enhancing its value.

Knowledge sharing takes place between two individuals; one possesses knowledge and the other acquires knowledge. In terms of the peer-led induction, given that the crucial endeavour is to offer reassurance, support and provide information, this should take place between management and staff, intra-staff, between staff and peer support workers and between staff/peer support workers and the mentees with this process involving the sharing of information, ideas, suggestions and experiences related to adapting to the new prison environment.

Implicit and explicit knowledge are the cornerstones of knowledge. In contrast to implicit information, which is difficult to share with others because it is very personalised, explicit knowledge is knowledge that can be communicated explicitly (Lai, 2013, p. 233). Explicit or tacit information can flow between people, or it can be used from others as groups, departments or organisations. Knowledge sharing refers to the voluntary activity by individuals to provide access to others to their own knowledge and experiences. The main processes of knowledge sharing in peer-led induction revolve around the transfer and dissemination of knowledge between individual and groups. Organisations identify knowledge sharing as a critical issue for a number of reasons, including the growing importance of the value of knowledge and the increasing recognition that tacit knowledge is more valuable than explicit knowledge (Marouf, 2007). Although knowledge is created and preserved by an organisation's employees, sharing knowledge with others requires a willingness to cooperate. As a result, sharing knowledge is not a simple procedure. Lack of information exchange can result in the dissemination of misleading, incomplete and inaccurate information, which is terrible for organisations (Zboralski, 2009).

A core and fundamental expectation is that the peer-led induction should actively facilitate and deliver information sharing. An overarching organisational principle is that 'sharing of information at the front-line level is essential in order to provide service users with the right support' (Curtis & Edwards, 2019, p. 355), and throughout the process of inducting prisoners, the peer-led induction should disseminate a range of information to achieve its aims and objectives. However, it goes beyond the simplistic notion of it being purely an information-sharing model as, by virtue of utilising peers and involving staff, it does in fact demonstrates attributes more akin to the concept of knowledge management and knowledge sharing. Such knowledge management is often viewed as an organisational process that covers the 'development, storage, retrieval and dissemination of information and expertise within an organisation' (Gupta et al., 2000, p. 3). The recognition of knowledge as a resource has become more prominent in organisational discourse, especially to ensure that it stays competitive and also innovative. Organisations have recognised the 'vast and largely untapped asset diffused around in the organisation knowledge' (Gupta et al., 2000, p. 4).

The transferable rationale behind the increased importance of knowledge organisationally is steeped firmly in the belief that effective management of knowledge brings positive outcomes that bring about institutional success. In fact, research evidence knowledge as the most crucial factor for success (Kogut & Zander, 1992; Nonaka & Takeuchi, 1995). Furthermore, effective and judicious use of knowledge also leads to increased productivity and performance (Asrar-ul-Haq & Anwar, 2016; Mesmer-Magnus & DeChurch, 2009). Knowledge that is not well managed and shared diminishes easily and rapidly. Knowledge sharing is naturally a related concept 'transference of knowledge among individuals, groups, teams, departments, and organizations' (Asrar-ul-Haq & Anwar, 2016). There are many factors that impact knowledge sharing practices, such as individual characteristics, as well as the characteristics of groups within the organisation. The organisation itself tends to affect the perspective of, and approach to, knowledge sharing. Cultures within groups, management and organisations as a whole interact with the individual and the values and norms associated with them and can influence the degree and flow of knowledge sharing (McKinnon et al., 2003). Knowledge management also fits within a managerialist rationale and approach to the peer-led induction. Some of the primary foundation behind it is the organisational need to be 'cost effective and managerially effective in problem-solving and decision-making', which is especially important to the prison in the era of do more with less (Gupta et al., 2000, p. 4).

Power is central to knowledge management and organisational learning (Engstrand & Enberg, 2020). The penal system reflects a post-structural Foucauldian power structure, where power is enacted through discursive behaviours – acting, talking and interacting – rather than being possessed (Foucault, 1977). It operates as a network of interactions, continuously in tension and activity. Self-techniques generate knowledge, reinforcing the relational nature of power

(Foucault, 1988). Power is both visible when exercised and diffused through institutional networks (Torfing, 2013; Townley, 1993).

Discursive positioning (Davies & Harré, 1990) builds on Foucault's concept of subjective positioning, framing the self as agentive and formed through relational interactions rather than socially determined (Winslade, 2005). In prisons, boundary work is crucial – how boundaries are enforced and how individuals position themselves within them directly affects the value of knowledge (Bucher et al., 2016). Institutional knowledge integration encounters syntactic, semantic and pragmatic boundaries (Carlile, 2002). Semantic boundaries, in particular, create conflicts over meaning, aims, values and alternatives (Von Meier, 1999). Pragmatic boundaries make knowledge political, as it becomes 'at stake' when embedded in specific roles and practices (Carlile, 2004). Negotiation of knowledge is thus shaped by power, which can enable or constrain participation in learning processes, as seen in peer-led induction (Contu & Willmott, 2023).

Investment in relationships, negotiation and coalition-building is crucial for knowledge integration (Faraj & Yan, 2009; Kellogg et al., 2006). While power in penal institutions is often perceived as negative (Lukes, 2005; Matthews, 2014), it can also be productive, shaping knowledge exchange through relational webs (Heizmann & Olsson, 2015; Marshall, 2006). Positioning theory highlights contradictions in knowledge integration – while integration literature often emphasises consensus, transformation emerges through tensions in discursive positioning. Boundary work allows institutional actors to 'establish, expand, reinforce, or weaken boundaries' (Zietsma & Lawrence, 2010). As such, border work in the prison setting can maintain or undermine discourse and infrastructure, resulting in negative impacts (Foucault, 1977).

Knowledge Conversion

For knowledge to truly realise its full value and to be harnessed to deliver its intended outcomes, especially in the case of peer-led induction, it must be effectively converted and transferred between individuals. Nonaka and Takeuchi (1995) demonstrate a typology of knowledge conversion with there being four processes, namely socialisation, capture, dissemination and internalisation: all relevant to peer-led induction although with variability in the level of relevance, implementation and actualisation.

Peer-led induction appears to follow some principles of 'Knowledge Conversion' (Gupta et al., 2000). This is firstly operationalised through the process of socialisation, whereby the interactive classroom-based induction components involve the sharing of experiences through observation, imitation and practice. There are a number of separate classroom and department-specific-based induction sessions that are employed in peer-led induction that cover various aspects of prison life. These sessions involve the sharing of information and experience regarding the function of these specific areas and their function. The general consensus among mentees was that the range and variety of information in this modular aspect to the peer-led induction was plentiful and delivered to them, which is a positive outcome. These supplement potential social interactions whereby information is shared. Conversations at the gym, at association, in the meal queues are all opportunities where peers and staff can socialise with those newly arrived prisoners.

Secondly, there is the conversion of tacit knowledge, from the domains of subjective, cognitive and experiential learning, such as the knowledge learnt in these classroom-based sessions into explicit knowledge in the form of written formats. Sometimes, prisoner mentees reported making notes while other preferred to supplement the interactive elements with the written information and forms that were issued during these sessions.

> There was a lot of information [...] too much to take in at times [...] I couldn't keep up. (Perry)

> I was trying to work out what I needed to prioritise when listening, but I couldn't so ended up getting proper worked up and flustered. (Peter)

There were, however, issues with these formats. A number of interviewees found that the number of sessions and the raft of information being presented to them were quite overwhelming and many found that capturing knowledge into explicit forms were difficult. Some of the interviewees expressed that this was due to low literacy levels while others cited attention deficits and difficulties being in the classroom/formal environment anxiety inducing in itself, due to these factors but also when coupled with lived experience of these settings in their formative years.

> There needed to be much more support [...] it was like we were invisible and so were they [mentors] [...] I was struggling and I felt isolated and on me own [...] they just weren't approachable or that interested. (Del)

The options to interact with mentors throughout the induction were viewed with caution by a substantial number of interviewees. There was the element of hierarchy that took place. Many interviewees viewed mentors as occupying a lofty position above them among the prison population. As such, mentees avoided approaching the mentors for help while others were met with an attitude from the mentors that symbolised them as being somewhat an inconvenience or irritant.

> It was like I was beneath them, an inconvenience [...] well, that's how I saw it anyways. (Joey)

Others simply stated that the mentors were just not visible to even approach. This undermines the full process of the peer-led induction if knowledge and information cannot be garnered. The confluence of principles, lived experience, context and insight that serves as the foundation for assimilating fresh experiences and knowledge (Gupta et al., 2000) are factors all undermined by the limited level of interaction.

The Prison Service Instructions (PSIs) governing induction goes on to state that all new prisoners must be provided with a booklet of '[e]ssential information about what will happen during their first few days in the establishment, and including information about the Samaritans, Listeners, Insiders, and any other peer supporter initiatives' (NOMS, 2015, p. 10). This pack or booklet should 'contain a brief description of what the prisoner can expect from their Offender Supervisor and clarify that they will be allocated an Offender Supervisor during their period in custody who will work closely with their Offender Manager in the community' (NOMS, 2015, p. 10).

This is a core component of prison induction with is entangled with the process of dissemination. This involves the conversion of tacit to explicit knowledge with this explicit knowledge disseminated through a range of materials both hard copy and digitally presented around the induction units, the departments and wings. This was largely present alongside socialisation in the induction intervention through the issue of induction packs and literature relating to the various areas and elements of the open prison establishment and processes.

> To be fair they did give us handouts to refer to and use which were pretty helpful to have a reference point. (Del)

> The leaflets with info helped me find my feet a bit by myself really which isn't a bad thing. (Paul)

While there may be deficiencies in the level of detail contained within the literature, in the level of their explanation and accessibility and the relevance of the information against needs, the provision of explicit knowledge does nonetheless take place. Furthermore, it is well received by a number of mentee interviewees who viewed them as a foundational offering in their adaptation to the new custodial setting. However, there was a more critical perception from some who viewed the level of dissemination as a way for staff and mentors to circumvent engagement with the mentees in the induction process. Rather than being a supplementary measure to underpin the peer support mechanism, they were in fact perceived as reducing peer support to a more subordinate role below the information handouts and as such limiting the role of peer support and the opportunity to engage with it.

Internalisation is the process of experiencing knowledge through an explicit source. In this sense, an individual can reconcile the experience of reading, listening and learning with that of prior experience. This knowledge internalisation, as the last stage, is key at the formative and transfer phases of knowledge transfer process but further at the knowledge promotion and application stage. It can be regarded as the reverse behaviour of the externalisation of tacit knowledge, inter alia, the implicitisation of explicit knowledge on the basis of innovation. In order to master a subject, knowledge subjects must first assimilate explicit knowledge into a higher level of tacit knowledge (Nonaka & Takeuchi, 1995). In the context of peer-led induction, success in this realm can be conceptualised with success measured twofold, as mentors reconcile these areas to deliver an effective intervention with mentees then being able to adapt and navigate the early days in the open establishment in a manner that does not exacerbate, and relieves, the pains of *entry shock* and *adaptation*.

PSI refer to a collection of policy documents that provide specific information about the rules, regulations and guidelines that must be followed in operational contexts. These are the primary legal documents that govern the prison system. The procedures to be followed are outlined in PSI 07/2015 (NOMS, 2015) with regard to being taken into custody, spending the first night in jail and the induction process. The governing PSI (NOMS, 2015, p. 9) states that prisoners must be placed on an appropriate induction and 'as far as possible, induction staff should confirm that prisoners understand the information they have been given and know where to seek further guidance'.

However, despite this key objective, unintended outcomes were often the reality:

> I was lost. I didn't have much idea about what was going on and I didn't feel I had the stuff I needed to figure it out [. . .] What I got was not what I needed and didn't answer the questions I had [. . .] questions went unanswered and led to more questions and this just got me worked up and ramped my anxiety up [. . .] It was testing. (Rich)

Prison Service Orders/Instructions clearly advance that 'Governors must ensure that all prisoners are given the information they need on the issues that are important to them' (NOMS, 2015, p. 2). However, the very use of peers to deliver induction, alongside staff, symbolises a more in-depth and complex notion than simply sharing information. Induction peer support workers, and also staff, should deliver knowledge, the core rationale for using them.

It is crucial to establish that knowledge is more than just information. Knowledge is 'information combined with experience, context, interpretation and reflections', a 'high-value form of information' (Davenport et al., 1998, p. 43). As Gupta et al. (2000, p. 17) state, it is 'an opportunity to find, select, organise and disseminate and transfer important information and expertise necessary for dynamic learning' with such learning being part of the wider induction process. Using peers to support and deliver induction allow the intervention to go beyond information sharing and foster experiential exchange with lived experience a vehicle for connect to allow for a more effective intervention to deliver better outcomes for those entering the prison environment. However, as Davenport et al. (1998, p. 43) have rightly recognised, while the motivation to create share and use knowledge is an intangible critical success factor for virtually all knowledge management, it is a complicated process to 'successfully transfer it from one person to another'.

There is the inference from the perception of staff and peer self-serving motives that these have had a detrimental impact on the induction process and are an indication of insufficient information sharing, as Joey claims:

> They're the ones who are set here [the mentors], they're meant to be helping us [...] they should know what we need [to know], but they don't give a fuck about telling us [...] guess that is cos they don't give a fuck about us or anyone but themselves.

A key challenge, therefore, to the management of the peer-led induction model appears to be, as Gupta et al. (2000, p. 19) recognise, 'how to convince, coerce, direct or otherwise get people to share their information'. This is especially relevant to staff whom are covered later in this chapter.

> They are there to help, right? All they ended up doing was ramping up my anxiety and stress. (Steve)

As has already been shown, the peer support workers may have information they could share with mentees who are exposed to the intervention but frequently decide not to do so. This is due in part to the motivational issues. It's possible that, content aside, there is a culture among peer support workers and, to some extent, the staff that lessens the efficiency of knowledge sharing and learning processes. It is to these and similar realities about knowledge sharing to which this chapter now turns and how they evidence induction as a tick box exercise.

The Pains of Transfer and Adaptation

> ...behaviour is situationally determined in the fullest sense of the concept, stemming from a complex of interactions between persons and environments at a given time. (Adams, 1992, p. 315)

Sykes (1958) introduced the notion of the pains of imprisonment as a deprivation thesis to explore how imprisonment is experienced by those subjected to it. A key foundation was that these psychological pains could serve to be more damaging than overt physical punishments. This was built upon by the theorisation of Foucault (1977), who considered that the replacement of this physical punishment may by a more civilised process yet more penetrative in nature. As already established the pains of imprisonment previously identified still exist institutionally, yet the reconfiguration of penal power has 'added an additional layer of frustrations' 'different in their sources, their feel, and their effects' (Crewe, 2011a, p. 512). These are neither an exhaustive nor exclusive set of pains that are experienced. The book proposes that limiting oneself to the narrow confines of Sykes and Crewe's pains neglects a range of other pains associated with differing aspects of the experience of imprisonment. Of the other 'forgotten' pains of imprisonment that have been identified, there are two especially pertinent to peer-led induction: *entry shock* and *adaptation*, with *adaptation* centring around *fear of the unknown*.

Entry shock is related to the tumultuous phase that those imprisoned navigate during their initial period of their imprisonment (Jones, 2007, p. 23). However, this can be extended to reception into any prison environment, whether from the community or being received after transfer from another establishment. At this juncture many prisoners can be overwhelmed by the imposition of a new regime and the change in their lived reality (Caird, 1974; Jones, 2007). It is evidenced that entering the criminal justice system can be a situation that underpins increased self-harm, suicidality and mental health issues, due to its disruptive and chaotic equilibrium distorting effect. This is especially true in the early days of custody. However, when considering the early days of custody, the stressor points of transfer between prisons and entry to a new establishment can also be included. Although literature suggests that the transition from freedom to prison is associated with the higher rates of self-harm and suicide due to it being more sudden than a transfer between incarceration, this does not mean that it is not still experienced acutely (Blaauw et al., 1998; Ingram et al., 1997; Jones, 2007).

> I didn't have a clue what to expect [. . .] you hear so many different things you just don't know what it's going to turn out like. (Peter)

> It was torture waiting [. . .] they don't tell you when you are going to transfer for security reasons so every day I was waiting for the knock on the door last minute to tell me to pack my stuff ready to transfer [. . .] I was living out of banana boxes packed with my stuff ready to go. (Jimmy)

In fact, when transferring from closed conditions to open conditions this can be a protracted process waiting for paperwork to be completed, signed off and computed, then waiting for transport booking and for spaces becoming available. Here, the suddenness is replaced by uncertainty and rumination that comes with awaiting the next step to freedom that you have been approved for a source of profound anxiety. A number of interviewees concurred with this position and said that waiting to transfer to open conditions was far worse an experience for them than entering custody from the community, and there was almost the presence as evidenced above of a 'pre-entry shock' as they prepared for the inevitable knock at the cell door to tell them they were transferring although when that knock would come was unknown and increased prisoner's anxieties.

The transfer to a new establishment also signifies that those imprisoned 'leave one world or life and enter another' (Jones, 2007, p. 25). Again, originally intended in relation to those transitioning from the community to custody, it can, however, be extended to inter prison transfer. A number of the interviewees had experienced a number of differing 'worlds' through the various prisons and associated regimes that they had experienced on their journey. In their early stage of transition, it can be said that there is evidence of liminality as prisoners hold on to aspects of their previous prison and regime while trying to acculturate to and reconcile their unfamiliar environment. At this point, as Harvey (2007, p. 31) muses that they 'neither relinquished their hopes from which they had been torn, nor yet accepted their existence within a new enclosed order'.

> Years of doing things one way, then bang it was turned on its head. Things were so different, I kept making comparisons to my old nick but they weren't the same [. . .] in hindsight I dunno why I did, they were totally different prisons, security, and all that [. . .] just putting more pressure on myself I guess. (Steve)

This is illustrative of *entry shock* when arriving at the prison, a theme that was shared almost unanimously among the ex-prisoner interviewees. Despite the fact that some interviewees had been in numerous prisons during their sentences and some had been in open prisons before and experienced the process of transfer, it still was a process and environment that caused acute feelings of fear and anxiety, arguably due to the ever-changing construct of the prison. The penal estate and the institutions within it are ever changing as a result of multiple dynamic factors, so the prison will always as a result be different every single time, inducing the state of fear. This then becomes a process, moving on to an early construct of *adaptation* founded upon an acceptance of the new situation and world within which prisoners find themselves within. As time goes by, this adaptation is elevated to the point where prisoners not only have better adaptation but they are also able to apply their adaptation to benefit from it (Harvey, 2007; Jones, 2007).

> I was scared shitless [. . .] I was trying to front it out, so no-one picked up on it, but just sitting in the reception I was totally on edge [. . .] things were about to change and the consequences of not getting it were gonna mess things up for me and my family. (Joey)

> I was so close, close to spending time at home with my family and getting back to normality [. . .] it was pressuring though cos I could see the high security prison across the road, and I knew I could end up back there at any point. (Peter)

The idea of liminality has been a theme, both in the experience of imprisonment and researching; however, there is room to further extend this notion by proposing the presence of a 'double liminality' whereby prisoners in the open prison do not just occupy a position between their former incarcerated world and present incarcerated world but also a position between the present occupied word and the free world. This 'double liminality' is especially acute given the prospect of a return to more onerous imprisonment or freedom. Applying the concept of double liminality to prisoners in open prisons offers a nuanced understanding of their psychological and social experiences. It highlights the compounded challenges they face as they manage multiple transitions, each requiring adaptation to new roles, identities and social norms. Liminality can intensify self-subjection by placing individuals in a state of uncertainty, instability and transition, where the rules are ambiguous and their future remains unresolved and even more compounded in the construct of double liminality where prisoners experience being caught between incarceration and release. The stakes are high, so this liminality certainly exposes why *entry shock* is as profound as the interviewees state, encapsulated in the quotes above.

> ...anxiety went sky high [...] I overthink at the best of times but new prison, new people, new rules, new things to learn it kind of takers over your thoughts. I was obsessing over it and it was stressing me out. (David)

Fear is a word that has been mentioned on a number of occasions so far and also by those interviewed. *Entry shock* does not exist on its own in the early days of experiencing a custodial setting, and it is associated with *fear of the unknown*, which is a particularly acute experience among those transferring and transitioning.

> I didn't know what was coming next [...] I had some ideas or guesses, but I weren't sure [...] that's a surreal and scary position [...] just not knowing. Waiting. (Freddy)

Fear of the unknown is arguably a manifestation of a lack of information that individuals are given in relation to the situation and environment that they find themselves in, and this was as evidenced above a common theme among those entering the open prisons into which they were received. Some of the underlying conditions for this fear resonate with the research of Jones (2007) who found that this was often the product of a criminal justice system interviewees were exposed to that kept them firmly shut out. In the prison environment, *fear of the unknown* is associated with uncertainty surrounding the prison itself, family ties and the liminality earlier introduced can exist inside a vacuum until adaptation is achieved. Liminality deepens subjection by creating a permanent state of uncertainty, where prisoners must manage their own compliance, regulate their behaviour and accept institutional narratives about their progress. This reinforces institutional power while masking coercion as self-determination, making freedom feel like another form of control. As such, pain continues to exist in the face of fear. However, as Adams (1992) asserts, prisoners have adjustment issues. Therefore, the ability to address this at the time when it is experienced most acutely, through intervention in the form of peer-led induction, is crucial in mitigating the pain experienced. All too often limited strategies for coping are offered or, as in the case of peer-led induction, when it is offered, it does not deliver what it should do to help those imprisoned adapt in a needs-driven manner. This is often due to it being undermined by responsibilisation, which is often perceived as a faux-motive for more sinister undercurrents surrounding staff motivations to help prisoners.

Establishing the Basics: Doing the Bare Minimum (at Best)

> As long as hit the first-night requirements that's the priority. (Officer Kev)

> We have to follow the guidelines as set down by the PSI and management. (Officer Woody)

The main result of the first night in custody is that 'prisoners are kept safe and supported during their first night in prison', as well as having their urgent needs handled, and this signifies the importance of supporting prisoner mental health and well-being. It continues to emphasise the severe trauma that offenders go through when ties to their families, communities and future are severed. As a result, focus is placed in custody on 'tackling safer custody difficulties during the first 24 hours and beyond is expected to yield maximum value in this early time' as 'many self-inflicted deaths and self-harm events occur between the first 24 hours, first week and first month'. Peer supporters 'may offer additional help to convicts, particularly during the first night' (NOMS, 2015, p. 7). Prison staff acknowledge this importance and focus as according to Officer Kev, as a prison officer involved in the induction process, 'The main thing is we check they aren't going to cut up or string up'.

> Prisoners assessed as being at risk of suicide or self-harm should have support identified and managed with all newly arrived prisoners assessed as part of the reception health screen process to determine whether they are at risk of suicide or self-harm. (NOMS, 2015, p. 13)

This is important as 'prisoners [. . .] are at increased risk of suicide/self-harm, and the risk occurs with transferred prisoners as well as those on initial reception into custody' (NOMS, 2015, p. 13). Staff members are therefore required to understand and abide by national and local guidelines on avoiding suicide and managing self-harm that are outlined in safer custody policies. Despite the fact that this assessment was always conducted, all participants described it as robotic process lacking fluidity.

> It was like a conveyor belt [. . .] one after the other, in and out job. (Steve)

Interviewees said that once staff members were confident they were not going to harm themselves or take their own lives, they moved on without addressing the causes of these manifestations, which included anxiety, stress and depression, all of which they self-reported having.

> I was so stressed [...] I told 'em but they said see healthcare in the morning and that it was just a bit of anxiety [...] I bet if I had told 'em I wanted to cut up they'd have paid attention. (Billy)

> They weren't interested in my mental health issues [...] I told 'em I was on meds, but they didn't wanna chat about that or how I felt- just if I had problems with self-harm and thoughts of suicide. (Webby)

It indicates that once the offender disclosed that they did not feel suicidal or motivated to commit self-harm, they were not given the proper consideration. Staff members are therefore required to understand and abide by national and local guidelines on avoiding suicide and managing self-harm that are outlined in safer custody policies. Despite the fact that this assessment was always conducted, all participants described it as a mechanical process.

Being in an open prison does not in itself mitigate or nullify the effects of imprisonment, and indeed, being an offender in the open estate comes with its own pains of imprisonment. The notion of *entry shock* and *pains of adaptation* are experienced most acutely at this juncture. However, again, the prison staff appeared to have little awareness of this acuteness and the wider range of its manifestations and sought instead to adopt a tick-box approach in relation to managing self-harm and suicidality, without exploring the mental health deficiencies that this manifest from.

> Support and guidance cost nothing, but it seemed to be a big thing to them [staff and peer mentors], no interest in me [...] couldn't even get the basics right [...] kick a man when he is already down was what it was like. (Jimmy)

It is widely acknowledged throughout the PSI that some prisoners received into prison 'will need support and assistance to resolve urgent and immediate issues arising as a result of their imprisonment and which adversely affect their lives (or the lives of others) outside the prison' (NOMS, 2015, p. 9). The PSI (NOMS, 2015, p. 9) states that the prison establishment needs to '[h]elp prisoners to uphold their immediate responsibilities to others by assisting them to solve immediate problems and make arrangements to cover the time they will spend in prison'.

For example, they may be worried about having left family members without an explanation of where they are. It states that during the initial interview:

> ...staff must take time to listen to prisoners and offer them help and support in resolving or managing their most urgent issues and in particular those that arise directly as a result of their imprisonment, time and resources must be available to resolve issues that cannot be left unresolved overnight and to provide personal help and support to prisoners as needed. (NOMS, 2015, p. 9)

> Ideally, we would like to spend more time with them and do more, but we just don't have the time [. . .] the best we can do is a quick first night interview to cover the basics that we have to do. (Officer Kev)

There was a sense of disinterest presented, but it was clear from the officers' responses that they felt they could, and would like to, do more but lacked the time to do so. As a result, they were forced to make do with a meagre offering that fell short of assuaging newcomers' worries and problems and of the level of support that both staff and inductees would hope for.

The PSI (NOMS, 2015) governing induction states that the expectation is that first night staff should be supported by Induction Insiders in this task. The peer support workers involved in the peer-led induction should shoulder the responsibility of being bound by the PSI directly or to ensure that mental health issues experienced by prisoners are addressed. This is the responsibility of prison staff who are involved in the induction process. However, there were alarming deficiencies in this area in terms of the support offered by peers to contribute to achieving the PSI.

> The peers couldn't wait to get me out the door so that they could crack on with cooking their dinner and playing pool [. . .] every time I asked a question they just fobbed me off and told I'd figure it out as I went along. . . (James)

> As soon as I signed their paperwork, they did a Houdini and vanished, and I never saw them again during the time I was on the induction wing. (Rich)

The comments above clearly indicate a distinct lack of interest from the peers in assisting with this process, and there was a prevalent perspective that the peers were only interested in having their paperwork signed off which indicates to others that they had 'done their job'.

The PSI states that:

> Equally, some prisoners may need additional support and assistance in understanding and adapting to the prison environment and that all prisoners new to custody and new to the establishment must be provided with key information relevant to their first few days in the establishment. (NOMS, 2015, p. 10)

The PSI also recognises that 'prisoners new to custody are likely to find the reception and first night periods confusing and even overwhelming, and that staff should try to help them settle in and overcome their anxieties' (NOMS, 2015, p. 7). It states that staff should also ensure prisoners are aware that safer custody is among the highest custodial priorities, with the responsibility of these measures being both effective and the establishment Governor's responsibility. It is apparent that the process and period of induction is identified and evidenced as being a difficult time for prisoners, with mental health and well-being issues and needs not being adequately addressed in the early stages of the peer-led induction, whether by the prison officers or those peer support workers supporting.

'We Seek Them Here, We Seek Them There' (Davies, 1966)

The formerly imprisoned interviewees, however, overwhelmingly agreed that staff and peers helping prisoners to acclimatise and settle to overcome anxiety was not the case. Although the officers and peers met with the mentees and ticked the box, the majority of those interviewed said that they did not disseminate the required information. Additionally, they stated that on the first night, both the peers and the induction staff did not adhere to these guidelines entirely. Others provided recollections of receiving piecemeal paper-based information, such as timetables for induction activities for the coming days, before being sent on their way. Many of these came with no explanation, and many of these sessions were reported later as not run-on time or even run at all.

Some reported only being told the roll call times and mealtimes and asked whether or not they had any thoughts of suicide and/or self-harm, signifying that these were the basics that were deemed necessary for a prisoners' immediate adaptation needs. In this context, the key concept is need and more accurately, unmet needs of those experiencing their adaptation to the new institution. It is clear that staff and peers once again carried out a meagre attempt to partially satisfy a guideline rather than implementing and delivering a needs-driven offering.

> Everyone is out for themselves [...] they ain't interested in helping us settle in and adjust [...] They are only interested in what suits them. (Rich)

All officers interviewed were vociferous in their presentation of heavy workloads and managerial pressure to meet guidelines, not only creating huge time constraints impacting the ability to do their job as they would like but also resulting in a culture whereby staff seemingly do everything by the book rather than using their professional judgement. It seems that the shackles of 'unhelpful' government targets and guidelines require the adherence to centrally prescribed ways of working, diminishing any prospect of local-level autonomy in aspects of the practice. However, as this chapter also identifies, there is a semblance of autonomy within the peer-led induction for staff to manage the process within the parameters of their management decreed focus. This begs the question of whether they could have actually done more?

> No time. They sit on their arse drinking coffee in the office. (Jimmy)

The majority of mentees interviewed definitely thought more could be done and expressed the perspective that officers and peers 'hid behind' the sentiment that they were tied down by paperwork and as a result, didn't have the time to deliver the intervention appropriately, when the reality was that, in fact, they preferred not to carry out their duties as prescribed.

Likewise, the peers delivering induction were eager to bemoan the volume of paperwork and the tick-box culture to mentees although again the consensus among the mentees interviewed was that they also hid behind this notion and demonstrated a lack of interest in the role they were supposed to be carrying out. As Rich says:

> There is a fair bit of info, but they aren't interested in going through it with you. They just want your squiggle [signature] to say you've read it and they are covered. (Rich)

The officers interviewed impressed the recurring sentiment that there was a distinct lack of time to focus on the care of transitioning prisoners. This is situated largely within a framework of the 'violence of austerity' with austere conditions and a lack of staff combined with a diverse set of offenders often presenting with complex needs and tremendous pressure from management to do more for less and comply with rules and regulations. These arguably culminate in culturing an environment and, more specifically, peer-led induction interventions that are devoid of being conducive with effectiveness and promoting positive well-being outcomes.

Given this much presented theme of a lack of time, it was not surprising that officers welcomed the use of peers leading the induction, although as this chapter later covers, this is not a unanimous consensus within prison officer culture. Staff interviewed actively 'contracted out' to peers on a regular basis, showing a willingness to share power for the purpose of managing their time more effectively but also to 'make things a lot easier for us' (Officer Emily). This resonates with the notions of prisoners becoming an in-situ institutional labour resource. Peer support workers/mentors effectively act as a diversion service on the frontline for dealing with prisoner questions and queries, thus allowing time for professional staff to be deployed in other areas of the prison and to do other duties in their role. What was clear was that there was a much greater focus and concern in relation to the day-to-day tasks associated with the running of the wing and prison generally rather than with the process of the induction programme and mentee needs. The pitfalls of power-sharing in this sense are that, even though the peer supporters become interred into the operational structure, it is compromised and a fragile proposition, given the almost careless delegation of such power to these peers. In this sense, the self-serving motivations of staff become the priority and result in what Crewe and Liebling (2017, p. 907) refer to as power being handed to peers in an 'informal, collusive and unaccountable' manner.

> The induction orderlies [peer support workers] run the show [. . .] The kangas [prison officers] let them do whatever they like, sort

> them out access to their property and treat them easier if they make their life easier and do what they should be doing. (Pauley)

There is the strong presence observed among the prison interviewees of prisoner hierarchy when it comes to the highly regarded roles in prison, such as peer support work. Seemingly, prisoners with the greatest level of credibility, influence and ingratiation among staff, and sometimes their peers, are perceived as attracting influential work placements. This is coupled with accompanying perks and benefits such as greater freedom of movement within the prison walls, greater access to staff, favourable parole reports and being shown in a favourable light with prison gatekeepers – these often offered in exchange for them exerting their influence over the new inductees, almost as a form of governance. These notions form the basis for mentors 'feathering the nest', whereby the true rationale for being a peer supporter is for self-serving motivations such as trafficking of contraband, extortion and bullying.

This is evidenced in the research findings through diminished staff authority, a steeper prisoner hierarchy and imbalances of power in the sharing initiative, all of which serve to re-enforce and exacerbate the triggers and stressors identified by ex-offender participants, creating the impression of what Dilulio (1987) terms a 'corrupt alliance'.

> You do not get any of the things you are really after, such as prisoner wellbeing and personal development, which we know are linked to all the outcomes we are interested in, until all the basic hygiene things, such as policing and security, staff professionalism, respect, humanity and safety, are in place. (Liebling, as seen on Parliamentlive.tv, 2017)

However, a range of underpinning factors permeate the intervention leading to this point. It is to these factors that the chapter now turns through the lens of Managerialism and Staff cultures.

A Recipe for Disaster: Managerialism and Staff Culture

Culture has been identified as a pivotal construct that can either enable or obstruct knowledge sharing and transfer (Asrar-ul-Haq & Anwar, 2016). Culture is 'a system of beliefs rooted in the society and expressed through the behaviour of the people and organizations' (Asrar-ul-Haq & Anwar, 2016). Culture is documented as a key factor in relation to knowledge sharing and knowledge transfer, in role as the precursor to knowledge sharing.

> They [management] tell, we do, it's that simple [...] they don't need us to help them with that. (Officer Kev)

That said, managerialist approaches of the prison institution to peer-led induction are an issue eroding the notion of a community culture. Such managerialism is described as 'a set of beliefs and practices at the core of which is the assumption that better management is an effective solvent' (Pollitt, 1993, p. 1). Deshpandé et al. (1993) explain community culture as a culture where the entire focus is on cohesiveness of employees rather than achieving goals. In this construct, employees participate in organisational decision-making, and their satisfaction is a key driver and consideration. This is sadly lacking in the case of peer-led induction, the officer sample expressing a lack of involvement in decision-making to the extent of being 'cut out' by management.

> It's about ticking the box for the things they focus on. Everything else is a free for all. (Officer Woody)

Staff perceptions seem to align with a perspective of management as one behind a bureaucratic culture; by focusing on the adherence to rules and procedures, it overlooks assets such as 'insights, intuitions, hunches, gut feelings, values, images, metaphors and analogies' (Nonaka & Takeuchi, 1995, p. 5). Literature (Asrar-ul-Haq & Anwar, 2016) has evidenced that such culture can have a positive relation with knowledge sharing behaviours. However, this is not the case in relation to the peer-led induction, especially when considering the relationship between management and staff. Officer Kev's comment is indicative of this:

> Why should I bother helping them? They don't give a shit and they treat us like shit so why help them?

Organisational culture has been recognised as a significant barrier to knowledge sharing by many (Asrar-ul-Haq & Anwar, 2016), acting as an omnipresent barrier to knowledge sharing and transfer in the institution as well as undermining the process of peer-led induction, given that prison officers are acknowledged as 'a diverse group, defending distinctly different visions and versions of the prison officer role' (Crawley, 2004, p. 168).

> The older staff who have been in the job for years are a bit more old school and don't like the new approach [...] they are more about giving out orders to people. (Officer Emily)
>
> When they [staff from other units] come onto the unit to cover, they are really dismissive of us and how we do things. They don't even make the effort to do things our way. (Officer Lily)

This signifies variability within the occupational group of the prison officers. They have a range of different attitudes, values and visions, and the comments from the staff interviewees are illustrative of what Crawley (2004, p. 188) conceptualises as 'pulling in other directions'. It is clear that there is resistance to the notion of power-sharing as this challenges traditional officer culture. Some officers create the impression that this sits outside their belief systems and attitudes to doing prison work; these are seemingly hard to relinquish when considering the staff interviewees comments. In this sense, they become fragmented as 'the old guard', 'which associated competence with masculinity, physical strength, and emotional toughness' (Crawley, 2004, p. 10). There is the notion from those staff interviewed that they saw these staff members as being aligned with Crawley's (2004, p. 9) description of being 'too disillusioned, too cynical, too frustrated, too frustrated or simply too old to buy into the organisations new ideal', in this case, the peer-led induction.

> Peer-Led Induction is about building relationships and rapport from our perspective [...] but other staff don't share that perspective. (Officer Emily)

Staff not sharing the ethos of a peer-led induction also undermines the value of establishing relationships. Within the notion of power-sharing and reconfigured penal power, there has been a shift to developing positive relationships between staff and prisoners moving away from historic adversarial approaches.

> There are some officers who don't get the changes [...] they think that they can do the induction without the use of prisoners [...] It's like they are a threat to them and the job. (Officer Emily)

> They [resistant staff] don't like that we talk to prisoners and aren't as full on [as them] [...] they seem to think that there needs to be a divide, like an us and them kind of thing. (Office Lily)

The comments above sit firmly in the realm of peer-led induction officers and the induction intervention running in ways that are 'contrary to the norm' (Crawley, 2004, p. 204). This means that interactions with prisoners deviate and depart from traditional institutional ethos and are met with resentment, antagonism and scepticism from officers failing to 'internalise and make it [power-sharing through induction] their own' (Gabriel, 1993, p. 135).

A theme emanating from the staff interviewees is that of openness to change, which is acknowledged as a fundamental cultural attribute behind the exchange of knowledge (Al-Adaileh & Al-Atawi, 2011). Openness facilitates effective communication in an organisation, and this can be extended to within intervention (Magnier-Watanabe, 2011). It is proffered that '[g]ood communication along with a climate of trust, openness, and sense of collegiality helps in the creation of an engaging environment that facilitates tacit knowledge sharing' (Nakano et al., 2013, p. 293). An issue that impacts the peer-led induction, however, is that when there is lack of time and workload is heavy, sharing and transfer of knowledge becomes difficult.

> We are flat out [...] there is so much to do and so little time, we have to make tough calls about what to prioritise [...] sometimes, well quite often, there are things we just can't do. (Officer Kev)

> If they [management] gave us proper resources we would be able to do everything that's needed, not just the things that get checked up on. (Officer Woody)

This can be situated within the notion that time pressure provides conditions that preclude knowledge sharing. Because of the violence of austerity within the prison estate, work pressure has also increased, which makes it difficult for prison staff to both involve themselves and do so effectively in knowledge sharing.

> I'd genuinely like to do more for them [prisoners], but my hands are tied. (Officer Emily)

Thus, heavy workload is a fundamental reason for having limited or no time for knowledge sharing. This issue around knowledge sharing is evident in staff-to-staff communication as well as staff-to-prisoner communication. The perception of staff and mentors engaged in this process is, however, one that is vastly different in the eyes of the ex-prisoner interviewees, as discussed earlier in the chapter. Even though both perspectives compete, what is unequivocal is that they are to the detriment of the peer-led induction intervention.

Both profit-making and non-profit organisations view performance as a critical issue. Increasing performance is something that most want to do. Several factors have been identified in the literature as having an effect on organisational performance and its improvement, including organisational culture, strategy, individual and organisational learning, employee involvement and commitment to organisational goals (Abu-Jarad et al., 2010; Bhatti et al., 2011; Uzkurt et al., 2013). Additionally, the non-economic facets of an organisation's social and societal interactions and competitive success elements that affect the effectiveness of its operations can be referred to as operational performance. Five criteria are typically used to evaluate operational performance: cost, quality, delivery, flexibility and innovation. These non-financial metrics are well-liked because they may be utilised to convert a strategy and vision into a tool that affects performance and produces superior performance.

Management support has been shown in research into knowledge sharing and transfer 'as a motivator or enabler of knowledge sharing' (Asrar-ul-Haq & Anwar, 2016, p. 10) with support stemming from management having a profound impact on knowledge sharing in practice (Cavaliere et al., 2015). Management leadership has a pivotal role in the promotion of knowledge sharing and transfer in any organisation, and the prison is no different. Central to the role is the ability to nurture and develop trust among employees as well as promote them to share and exchange their knowledge. Unfortunately, there was a lack of trust in prison management evidenced by the staff interviewees. Rivera-Vazquez et al. (2009) identify that management can take the form of a cultural barrier to knowledge sharing. Such a lack of trust has been identified as the biggest barrier that inhibits sharing of knowledge with others in the organisation (Asrar-ul-Haq & Anwar, 2016).

> They just want to hit their targets [...] that's their concern.
> (Officer Kev)

The staff interviewees indicated the perception of self-serving and selfish motivations of management rather than demonstrating effective leadership. As considered in Chapter 4, less pressure on staff resources can support management to meet their targets, with reducing staff workload also aligned with reductions in staff turnover, and a more cost-effective and captive workforce than that of utilising paid staff. Effective leadership enables knowledge sharing and transfer organisationally. However, the combination of deficient management support and poor leadership have hindered the successful sharing and transfer of knowledge in the prison environment. This has led to a gulf in knowledge especially in relation to the design, implementation and evaluation of the intervention, which feed into issues in the peer-led induction in these areas. As identified by McNichols (2010), lack of top management support acts as a barrier to knowledge sharing and transfer. There is a lack of focus on the individual as people with differing attributes that are all essential to the success of the institution and the mechanisms of the institution. This creates major problems to 'convince, coerce or direct people to share their information' (Gupta et al., 2000, p. 10).

On the other hand, poor leadership acts as a barrier to knowledge sharing and transfer. There is also a lack of motivation in the construct of recognition, praise and incentivisation that encourages the knowledge sharer to disseminate their knowledge to others (Gururajan & Fink, 2010). According to Dysvik et al. (2013), employees who voluntarily participate in the process of knowledge donation are more likely to be recognised for their efforts and intellectual capital, which in turn facilitates their managers' attempts to gather information. Additionally, participating in the process of knowledge donation can be crucial for organisations since it enhances their knowledge base by gradually changing individual information into collective and organisational knowledge (Alhady et al., 2011).

Just like prisoners are incentivised to display certain behaviours and practices, the same can apply to staff to support the transfer of knowledge to ensure the intervention is in an optimum state and to overcome some of the managerialist issues that are to its detriment in relation to management and staff relationships. However, this is sorely lacking.

> I do what their priorities are [...] that way I can't be criticised.
> (Officer Kev)

Staff also evidence a culture of fear and ambivalence towards management, and this transcends into the peer-led induction which itself is seen as aligned with managerialist strategy. The unrelenting top-down pressure of managerialist demands has resulted in staff being rigid and not prepared to deviate beyond these constraints. This is a sign of a high level of uncertainty avoidance in the prison, which is measured by how reluctantly individuals embrace ambiguity and uncertainty. People are more risk-averse and inclined to accept and adhere to norms, policies and laws inside the institution under this high uncertainty avoidance culture. The managerialist approaches stifle the 'wriggle room' for staff to be more entrepreneurial in some respects of the peer-led induction. Intolerance to new ideas and behaviours is also a key component of this and can be evidenced with the staff not embracing their reconfiguration of penal power through the power-sharing of peer-led induction.

However, there is a lack of balance as there is some evidence of staff having freedom within the intervention to develop it and construct it. In effect there is a structure within a structure, with staff evidencing high uncertainty avoidance stemming from top-down approaches and towards the managerialist peer support intervention and those associated with it. Yet, they are also able to evidence some semblance of low uncertainty avoidance through them being able to have more individualism when the time and resources allow and when they do not clash with management priorities. This low certainty avoidance in the context of peer-led induction is, however, fraught with issues surrounding inconsistency and variability in design, implementation and delivery, which may not be conducive with delivering the intended outcomes of the intervention. In fact, this process of assembling the peer intervention and its content from a perspective of what staff and peers deem 'is best' or 'what prisoners need' symbolises a lack of connection with input from those that matter, the prisoners coming into contact with the intervention. The lack of evaluation that permeates the peer-led intervention is indicative of this and leads the intervention to deviate away from a 'needs-driven model'. Given the findings applicable to the peer-led induction, it is important to consider the question posed by Curtis and Edwards (2019, p. 358), regarding intervention design; 'for whose benefit is this service intended?'. It is argued that 'the least successful [information sharing initiatives] have been those designed and imposed from a central bureaucratic perception of the needs of individuals and those committed to assisting them' (Curtis & Edwards, 2019, p. 358). There have been numerous examples from those interviewed which categorically and unanimously indicate that this is indeed the case and that the induction model falls within this category and is far from a needs-driven model.

> I'm not saying that they didn't think it was the right stuff [information], but it wasn't what I needed, what I wanted it more importantly when I needed it [...] it was more suited to them [staff and mentors]. (Peter)

It has been acknowledged that teams 'fail to share information when they most need to do so' and 'deviate from the optimal utilization of information' (Mesmer-Magnus & DeChurch, 2009, p. 525) despite it being a crucial aspect of any intervention success and 'serve to strengthen individual preferences rather than share correct information' (Mesmer-Magnus & DeChurch, 2009, p. 544). The mentee interviews, as illustrated above, expressed that this is apparent when providing information to those subject to the induction process.

The formerly imprisoned participants all expressed that they believe the available induction model is not one that is appropriate for needs-driven induction, and that the lack of pertinent information and content coupled with an inappropriate delivery has only served to increase anxiety and negatively affect their well-being during the transition to the establishment.

> It just made me more worried [. . .] I had a head full of questions I couldn't answer or get answered [. . .] I just wanted to say fuck it and do nothing. (Ally)

> All the years of jumping through hoops, kissing arse, going against everything I'm about to get here for my family and it was being threatened at the first stage. (Rich)

This sits in stark contrast to the intended outcome of the induction intervention. The governing PSI (NOMS, 2015, p. 7) advances its ultimate aim as being for '[p]risoners receive the relevant Induction to Custody package at a time and in a manner relevant to their individual needs' and also that '[p]risoners know and understand their entitlements and responsibilities, and how to access support and facilities available to them' (NOMS, 2015, p. 13). The current offering clearly falls down and fails to meet these aims. The peer-led induction needs to take the form of a collaborative endeavour, tailored to needs, not to belief and wishful thinking, between the mentees on one hand and the staff and peer support workers on the other.

> They need to sit down with us and ask us what would help us settle better [. . .] if they did that and gave us what we wanted to know then I would have felt so much better. (Rich)

> It's a great idea in principle, but they ain't got it set up right here to do that's all. (Steve)

> If they did what we needed then it would be really helpful. (Rich)

As the above show, despite the dominant negative discourse towards the model offered at the establishments, there are also pockets of positive aspects that have arisen from the empirical investigation of it with offender interviewees all expressing the idea that peer-led induction does have the potential to work. The challenge being, how to convert this potential. The portrayal of the establishment is one that lacks a responsive needs-driven approach to its processes and are led by a 'tick-box' mentality. Interviewees create an impression of rigidity rather than fluidity. This is through the institutional focus on compliance within a rigid set of rules. It does so through what Adams et al. (2006) describe as an 'Oppressive Attention to Marginal Detail', which challenges the notion of delivering intended positive outcomes for those subject to the intervention. This adherence hinders the cultivation of a more positive culture and a needs-based model, promoting the best outcomes for those imprisoned. The ex-prisoner participants all repeatedly identified the factors of distance from family, safety in the new establishment, uncertainty over regime and protocols within the new establishment, and lack of support and information as stressors triggering elevated levels of anxiety and insecurity impacting their functionality and general wellbeing. They were unanimous in calling for the implementation of an induction model focused on being tailored to individual needs. However, such a model is not evident in the Peer-Led Inductions experienced by the participants. What becomes apparent is that the central proposition of using peers and staff to support is being largely diminished by the pervasive nature of a tick-box culture and self-serving motivations which increase the psychological onerousness and ontological insecurity of prisoners and leaving them feeling like they are 'swimming in a shark tank' (Crewe & Liebling, 2017).

At present, the 'tick-box culture' means there is too much emphasis on following guidelines and rules instead of actually helping the prisoners transitioning into the prison in a more needs-focused manner. It means that the system is full of people 'doing things right' rather than 'doing the right thing' (2010). A plethora of relentless top-down targets and too many forms and procedures are preventing prison staff from providing transitioning prisoners the help they need and assessing whether that help has made a difference. As it stands, a 'one size fits all' approach appears to be in place. This reduces the autonomy of the induction staff and peers and fails to allow staff to think for themselves or to deliver a needs-driven model for induction.

What is clear is that there are severe deficiencies in a number of clear areas relating to the management and sharing of knowledge. There is a lack of clear purpose between management and staff, between staff, and between staff/peers and mentees. Underpinning this is a wholesale lack of a knowledge-friendly culture permeating through all echelons of the institution, often stemming from a lack of senior management support and trust in management. Resistance to change in the face of established occupational cultures and questionable motivations from staff and prisoners also undermine the intervention as well as narrow channels for knowledge transfer. All of these areas are core conditions for success in knowledge endeavours. All of them have profound shortcomings, which render the ability for knowledge to support delivery of the intended outcomes as a largely fruitless endeavour. The 'tick box' way, in which peer-led induction is operationalised, delivered and power-applied, means that it does not meet prisoner mental health needs and support positive outcomes. Intent in this instance does not lead to intended outcomes but instead lays a foundation for the unintended outcomes that arise as a result. The next chapter travels beyond the surface level expressions and considers more intricate arguments about the principles of peer-led induction being potentially quite problematic because they are infused with responsibilisation and managerialist cultures.

Chapter 6

Responsibilisation: 'It's Not Really What It Says on the Tin'

> Congratulations. You have survived the war. Now live with the trauma. (Lori Jenessa Nelson, n.d.)

The chapter signifies that peer-led induction extends beyond simply inadequately addressing prisoner metal health and well-being needs at the time of transfer, transition and adaptation to open prison. Instead, it is arguably indicative of making issues in these areas worse. It considers in what ways and to what extent do power-sharing initiatives impact the tightness of imprisonment. In doing so, it evidences the omnipresence of the diffuse concept of tightness at a number of junctures, and how it is experienced, in relation to wide ranging issues surrounding the concept of 'purported' responsibilisation, which is a strategy employed in the open prison estate. It does so through consideration of visibility and engagement of the staff and peers involved in the peer-led induction intervention and how it is both operationalised and experienced.

The chapter firstly introduces the notion of responsibilisation that has become a staple of prison strategy and policy in the contemporary prison. As Rose (1996, p. 59) states, 'the regulation of conduct becomes a matter of each individual's desire to govern their own conduct freely in the service of the maximization of their happiness and fulfilment that they take to be their own'. It advances responsibilisation as a strategy of self-regulation and governance through 'technologies of the self' in order to achieve both prison and individual objectives. A key factor experienced by those entering a new custodial establishment is stress, defined as a 'mentally or emotionally disruptive or disquieting influence' (Adams, 1992, p. 282). Prison reception is synonymous with elevated levels of maladaptive behaviours, which is a clear indicator of transition as a stressful experience. Adams (1992, p. 346) states that:

> Early research on prison adjustment focussed attention on attitudes during the middle stage of the prison term, or the point at which it was hypothesized that the influence of the prison

Navigating Mental Health in the Male Open Prison, 111–125

doi:10.1108/978-1-83549-706-720251006

> culture is the greatest and the influence of the community weakest. We now see that the beginning and the ending points of the prison term are critical transition periods when dealing with issues of stress and maladaptive behaviour.

He goes on to further state that previous research on prison adjustment also:

> ...clearly indicates a need for programs that help inmates to develop their coping abilities early in the prison sentence. These programs could use a variety of behavioural, cognitive, and social skills techniques to teach inmates to respond more effectively to difficult situations. (Adams, 1992, p. 345)

Peer-led induction is illustrative of the notion from Adams (1992, p. 345) that '[w]hen directed at problems of adjusting to prison life, such programs are likely to be effective and can bring immediate payoff'. The chapter therefore considers the role of peer-led induction and what it should deliver alongside its interaction with responsibilisation, which is perceived as a catch-all phrase to mask visibility of staff and peer support worker in the process and their lack of engagement with those inductees new to the prison. This is illustrative of failing to employ a needs-driven approach to induction. It considers how this 'perverse responsibilisation' interacts with the mental health and well-being of prisoners and is to their detriment.

It proceeds to consider how responsibilisation interacts with the notion of 'tightness', exploring how tightness 'captures the feelings of tension and anxiety generated by uncertainty, and the sense of not knowing which way to move, for fear of getting things wrong' (Crewe, 2011a). It considers how this is experienced through the fear of regression and a lack of progression in the open prison and how this fear is stoked by the peer-led induction. It signifies how responsibilising measures are experienced against a coercive backdrop, whereby this culture of fear is further re-enforced, culminating in unremitting distress. There are a number of competing themes and tensions that run throughout the consideration of responsibilisation. Theoretically, it is associated with aims to empower and enable, yet it in fact results in disempowerment and disabling effects underpinned by disinterest. Arguably, the overarching notion is that responsibilisation, whether it be genuine or employed as a buzz word to mask deficiencies within the programme, undermines the function of peer-led induction, promoting an existence fraught with tension, stress and anxiety among prisoners entering and adapting to a new custodial setting.

Responsibilisation

> ...from a variety of direction, the disadvantaged individual has come to be seen as potentially and ideally an active agent in the fabrication of their own existence [...] And, thus it follows, that they are to be assisted not through the ministrations of solicitous

> experts proffering support.. .. . .but through their engagement with a whole array of programmes for their ethical reconstruction as active citizens. (Rose, 1996, p. 60)

It is argued that crime control institutions have repeatedly failed to achieve their manifest goals (Foucault, 1977). Institutions for criminal law enforcement and punishment often fail to show that they do adequately, in fact, control crime, deliver justice and deliver care, but the problem is not merely that the apparatus of 'criminal justice' fails to work; in some instances, the mechanisms it introduces to do so produce outcomes that demonstrably make things worse. In the context of peer-led induction, this was encapsulated by Joey who states:

> It made shit worse [. . .] my head was ruined [. . .] I had so much shit going on and I was wobbling hard [. . .] New nick, new people, new things [. . .] it just made things go from 0 to 100mph in no time.

A Foucauldian perspective of governmentality has led to literature exploring the manner in which modalities of exercising and applying power are dependent on ways of thinking and ways of acting and, of central importance, 'ways of subjectifying individuals and governing populations' (Garland, 1997, p. 174). In this sense, 'the state alone is not responsible for preventing and controlling crime' (Garland, 1996, p. 453). This was extended out to the prison environment with literature documenting the offender's responsibility for their actions (Hinds & Grabosky, 2010; Matthews, 2005). As Hannah-Moffat (2000, p. 514) states, 'the state seeks to bring about action [. . .] either by simulating new forms of behaviour or by stopping established habits' on the part of the individual, in this case the prisoner. This leads to 'government at a distance' through 'a new mode of governing [offenders] with its own forms of knowledge, its own objectives, its own techniques and apparatuses' (Rose & Miller, 1992, cited in Garland, 1996, p. 454).

Responsibilisation symbolises the governing prisoners are no longer the sole responsibility of the government and prison but rather that of the offender themselves (Hannah-Moffat, 2000). Individuals, not government or institutions, are now responsible for their own destiny, their welfare and the consequences of their decision-making processes. Garland (1996) asserts that government commit resources on tough penal measures as a strategy of reasserting sovereign power to punish and in doing so, demonstrate ability to inflict harsh forms of punishment. In the contemporary prison estate, the government still asserts its power to punish. However, austerity extends to the prison estate, which lacks the resources and the historic mechanisms of punishment. As such, there is the necessity to do more with less, a recurring theme of this book.

Rose (2000, p. 334) notes the aim of responsibilisation to 'reconstruct self-reliance in those who are excluded'. This also allows them to gain an understanding of the 'values and ideas about the desirable attributes for taking part in society' (Ballesteros-Pena, 2018, p. 459), in this case the prison society. As Rose (1996, p. 59) states, 'the regulation of conduct becomes a matter of each individual's desire to govern their own conduct freely in the service of the maximization of their happiness and fulfilment that they take to be their own'. By engaging in peer-led induction, mentees are accepting responsibility in the eyes of the prison and as an understanding of what they need to do to govern themselves. Technologies of the self are the 'actions and strategies implemented in order to shape the individual and collective capacities of action in ways that are consistent with the objectives pursued by government in the neoliberal era' (Ballesteros-Pena, 2018, p. 458). It is postulated that these mechanisms of self-governance are implemented through a responsibilising process (Garland, 1997; O'Malley, 1999). The prison estate, and more specifically open prisons, use responsibilising governance in order to regulate and maintain order, 'producing a rational subject, self-governed and self-sufficient' (Ballesteros-Pena, 2018, p. 459). In the open prison, this is at its most acute. Here prisoners are the lowest risk prisoners, close to release, housed in institutions with low security and low staffing where freedom is consumed daily. The low staffing and security mean that prisoners subject themselves to their own form of governance, a disciplinary gaze upon themselves to compartmentalise freedom and temptation to gravitate towards what is mandated by the prison (Crewe & Ievins, 2020).

A Relationship of Inconvenience

After reviewing the prior evaluation of the Insiders Induction Scheme, it evidences a limited Programme Theory. When considering the earlier literature, there appears to be two key aims in relation to the use of peers in the peer-led induction:

(1) To offer reassurance to new prisoners and
(2) To provide them with key information that will be useful to them in their early days in custody (HMPS: Safer Custody Group, 2005).

It is an active form of peer support in terms of its objectives, function and operation when compared with more passive schemes involving the use of peers such as the Listeners, which was introduced in the earlier literature review chapter documenting peer support. In a peer-led induction model, the peer support workers do not have any expectation to provide emotional support nor do they receive any training to do so. They also do not have confidentiality principles to follow.

The perception of staff and peer support workers engaged in this process is, however, one that is vastly different in the eyes of the ex-prisoner interviewees. There is the perspective from the majority of interviewees that 'laziness' was the motivation behind extolling virtues of 'responsibilisation' on those seeking support.

> I'm all for being left alone to do stuff [. . .] but I still needed some support and information to get me to the point where I could, and I didn't get it [. . .] they were too busy sitting in the office. (Del)

> By far a bunch [the prison officers] of selfish, lazy cunts [. . .] doing the minimum. (Rob)

This resonates with research from Crawley (2004, p. 188) who describes 'lazy staff' as those who 'hide when undesirable jobs need doing...and who fob off prisoners seeking help'. This serves to undermine the relationships between staff and prisoners which documented as being at the centre of the functioning prison (Crewe, 2011b). However, intra-staff relationships also are negatively impacted by a lack of a shared sense of direction. Some of the officers interviewed described the performance of staff as not conducive with delivering the aims and ethos of induction (Crawley & Crawley, 2007). Coupled with the levied perception of laziness, this made the lives of prisoners and the enactment of the prison officer role in the context of induction more difficult and stress inducing. This notion of no shared sense of direction also plays out when considering the intra-staff relations explored within occupational staff cultures. Just as Crewe and Ievins (2020) identify, staff involved in the key decisions in the open prison around functions such as release on temporary licence (ROTL), Paid Work, Community Work and Community Engagement were simply unavailable and as a result are 'distant and under-informed' (Crewe & Ievins, 2020, p. 57) when it comes to actually making decisions relating to these areas. Here, they demonstrate absence and a lack of 'grip':

> They think we are stupid [...] none of 'em [peers] give a shit, not really, they're just looking out for themselves. (Peter)

> We've all got an agenda [...] theirs is just a bit more obvious than they'd like. (Joey)

The relationships between all parties involved in the peer-led induction are complex, and central underlying factors of any success must centre on using the principles of approachability, decency, stability and legitimacy. Interpersonal contact with staff was after all expressed by Lloyd (1990) as being the best countermeasure for those prisoners experiencing suicidal tendencies. However, they are based on what Crewe (2011b) terms as non-normative motives as the quotes above symbolise, with the process of mutual compulsion, a transactional mode of interaction pervading. Any interaction can be situational within theorisation that they are artificial in nature, based upon self-interest as much as a legitimised and genuine interaction. When combining instrumental interactions with a lack of genuine intentions alongside responsibilisation strategies, they have the effect of drawing the prisoner mentee away from interaction and accessing and establishing positive relations. As Bosworth (2007, p. 76) muses:

> Each articulation of power of the prison paradoxically undermines and reinforces the broader view [...] that prisoners act rationally [...] fully responsible for their actions. The threat of sanctions makes it all the more necessary for inmates to monitor their behaviour [...] reminding them that they are constantly under review.

What should be an endeavour to support autonomous individuals within the prison through peer-led induction actually creates an environment of dependence. The sufferings within the walls of the prison have not evaporated because of softening penal power through responsibilisation and the usage of peers. Even while some interviewees argued that the idea of responsibilisation is welcomed, it remains that all participants overwhelmingly agreed that it was improperly operationalised and that there was an excessive amount. As a result, these pains of imprisonment still exist and have changed in response to establishment-specific pains at the local level and are characterised by a tick-box culture. All of the offenders who were interviewed spoke about the negative effects of issues such as being stripped of their freedom, staff members abusing their power, other prisoners acting threateningly, the breaking of family ties, 'unremitting loneliness' (Johnson & McGunigall-Smith, 2008), the crushing of one's emotional existence (Jewkes, 2005a, 2005b) and 'institutional thoughtlessness' (Crawley, 2005).

> My head was a mess [. . .] I just wanted to go back [. . .] I was up the creek without a paddle. (Joey)

> I was struggling mate [. . .] fuck me [. . .] I thought I was passed being scared but here I was the same guy who can't deal with his shit [. . .] Sounds absolutely pathetic but it's how I felt [about trying to adjust]. (Steve)

It is further argued that by responsibilising offenders, it also allows staff and peers the time to fulfil their self-serving motivations and/or observe the tick box and 'arse-covering' culture discussed. They also reported a distinct lack of support again based upon the assumption of tacit knowledge about the prison due to having been in custody in other establishments. As Steve notes:

> You've been in a few times so long enough to know how to do your bird you'll pick things up quick was the great advice from the mentors. (Steve)

> I've been in high security for years where you get told what to do and when nothing happens without asking someone first and then you wait and fucking wait [. . .] I've rocked up here and it's the other way, and it's hard to adjust [. . .] but they can't see that- they think it must be easy to go from one extreme to the other, but the thing is [. . .] year after year after year that was my life and routine- being here don't mean I'm gonna adjust overnight- it needs time and a little bit of help. (Sammy)

However, this is a dangerous assumption as further reported conditions across establishments vary, and dynamics of prison life differ on all levels and are experienced differently depending on each prison's context as established earlier when considering the pains of entry and adaptation.

> Whenever the screws and peers couldn't be arsed to answer a question or help out or do something for me they just kept saying it was up to me to find out, or it was my responsibility to find out/sort it [...] but if I knew how or if they had told me things I needed to know then I wouldn't have asked in the first place! (Pauley)

> You need to start doing things for yourself [...] you're gonna be going on day release in the community soon and you ain't gonna have no-one to wipe your arse for you then, that was the excuse they kept giving me not to do shit. (Steve)

These quotes above encapsulate an almost perverse form of responsibilisation. This attitude purports to an attempt to enable and empower the prisoner, when in fact many interviewees felt it was an all too convenient excuse not to maximise the benefit of induction and provide the much-needed support. Instead of giving their time, knowledge, information and support, it allows them, namely the peer supporters and prison induction staff, to 'pass the buck'. This purported responsibilisation of prisoners sits in direct contrast to a fundamental purpose and spirit of the induction process of reducing anxiety and promoting well-being. Instead, it especially underpins the pains of self-governance and also those associated with transfer, transition and adaptation. Such strategies of responsibilisation delegate 'coordination, control and surveillance onto inmates' (Ballesteros-Pena, 2018, p. 473). It signifies a managerialist approach of governance that should allow for a more efficient and performance achieving construct. However, the reality is quite different. Here the contradictory nature of power plays out in the open prison and exemplifies the tension between care and control.

This also aligns with the issue of officers lacking the means to help provide a clear path for prisoners that makes the things required of them attainable and clear. The Prison Service Instruction (PSI) mandates that '[I]nformation is provided to prisoners. Prisoners are aware of how to use the resources and services offered to them in this facility' (NOMS, 2015, p. 7). Despite this goal, every prisoner interviewed expressed fear and worries about bullying and safety in the new facility and was actively looking for assistance and reassurances that these worries were unfounded. They did, however, emphasise that they didn't get these.

> A big concern for me was bullying and violence. I know there aren't many guvs about [...] I was told that violence wasn't a big issue and if I had any concerns to go see a rep [...] end of [...] no information to reassure me about why it isn't a problem or how they deal with it [...] Prison is full of vultures so to go speak to a rep who is a prisoner and tell him I'm scared and vulnerable and share my personal shit made me really anxious. (Joey)

When considering the adjustment issues that are connected to self-injury and mental disorder, they have been largely associated, especially by Toch (1975, cited in Adams, 1992, p. 288) as efforts to 'alleviate themselves of severe emotional distress'. Adams (1992, p. 288) extends Toch's ideas to identify that prisoners therefore can turn to coping strategies that involve:

> ...classifying themselves as victims, and make clear to staff their inability to deal with this status [...] also may enlist the assistance of staff in trying to deal with their difficulties [...] convince staff to be placed in a specific prison environment or setting [...] or demands on staff.

Although being granted a semblance of autonomy and choice under the guise of 'responsibilisation', as Giddens (1991, cited in Crewe, 2011a, p. 519) carefully observes, 'the prisoner is exposed to a greater degree of risk.... this opening up of possibilities, however narrow, provokes feelings of anxiety and powerlessness'. This is evidenced in the following quotes:

> What's the point of having peers and staff if they ain't gonna help? [...] It just stressed me out even more. I didn't know what to do or how to go about doing it when I did [...] just made everything so fucking hard. (Alan)

> Peer support was a myth [...] in a strange environment after years in a different nick, and I was told to crack on with it and figure things out myself [...] I just wanted to go back [to my previous prison] amongst what I knew [...] I was stressed to fuck by it all. (Steve)

That said, many prisoners have adjustment issues. Therefore, a problem with responsibilising strategies is that '[they] are poorly situated to participate in correctional programs and can drain institutional resources by consuming inordinate amount of staff attention' (Adams, 1992, p. 276). Some of the officers interviewed reported prisoners having such adaptation issues; however, their approach was naive. They were rather one-dimensional in their assessment, seeing prisoners as a drain on their time instead of recognising the complex history of those coming into contact with them. There is variability as such in the institutional environments where prisoners have previously been located, with some prisoners adjusting better in some settings than others, while others have adjustment difficulties at various stages of their life and indeed sentence.

> I guess I was wrong about us being in it together [prisoners] [...] there weren't no community, just individuals focussing on what was in their best interests. (Freddy)

The awareness of variability was in lacking consideration and empathy, among staff but also among the peer support workers. Those very people who were supposed to be supporting their fellow prisoner were perceived as viewing these individuals as in some way being an inconvenience and an unwelcome imposition. This is a clear early indication that what should be an altruistic endeavour is deficient in this area and potentially indicates self-serving motivations as a primary driver of those involved in the induction process. It also serves to disrupt the adjustment process, which Clemmer (1940) terms 'prisonization', whereby the prisoner assimilates themselves into the prison population and community. The 'individual differences in perceptions, needs, skills and abilities are seen as critical factors in adjustment', according to Adams (1992, p. 282). However, the institution fails to recognise them.

It is not to say that prisoners to do not attempt to engage in responsibilising themselves. Even when they do try to use initiative in the face of an ineffective induction model that lacks responsivity to need, they get stuck in a perpetual cycle of responsibilisation where being responsible is met by responses to be 'responsible'. All of this leaves an enduring stain from the pain of imprisonment associated with *entry shock* and *adaptation*.

Treading on Eggshells: The Fear of Regression and (or) Lack of Progression

The study indicated that the most appropriate metaphor to characterise the impact of the responsibilising nature of the induction is arguably that of 'tightness' rather than 'weight'. 'Tightness' is an aspect of the multifaceted concept of 'weight'. However, 'the shape and distribution of the penal burden have shifted, like a sack of sand remoulding itself across the body of its bearer. There are more levers of compliance and regulation, and therefore, more points where the weight is felt' (Crewe, 2011a, p. 524). It appears that while the pains of imprisonment can be reduced to some degree, pain is intrinsic and will merely manifest in alternate forms and different contexts as a result of different applications of power and operationalisation, rather than being eliminated from the prison experience. As Crewe (2011a, pp. 512–513) muses, the reconfiguration of penal power in prisons in England and Wales has 'worked alongside established pains in determining the experience of imprisonment, but they are different in their sources, their feel and their effects'. Power in this context, as applied by the induction prison staff and peer support, 'does not so much weigh down on prisoners and suppress them' as engulfing and smothering them, coercing them to conduct themselves in particular ways (Crewe, 2011a, p. 522).

> They are on top of you all the time [...] just waiting to fuck you over. (Rich)
>
> You have to do it one way or the other. (James)

This 'tightness' described here is the epitome of anxiety, stress and tension. Prisoners feel rudderless, trapped in inertia for fear of moving in the wrong direction and getting something wrong. It is connected to the acute tensions and insecurity that are experienced when a prisoner is fearing a regressive move or a lack of privilege or progression in the prison environment. Crewe (2011a) states that this is a normative companion of therapeutic coercion; however, it also extends to intervention, such as peer-led induction, in an established associated with the lowest levels of security and highest levels of autonomy.

> I didn't wanna get anything wrong in case it stopped me getting my home leaves on time. I was constantly feeling like I was treading on eggshells, so I made the move to stay out of the way in my cell. (Harvey)

As such, the autonomy granted by the establishment to its population is limited and circumscribed, and power is tight because the 'smack of firm governance' is always waiting in the wings to make sure this autonomy is exercised in a proper manner (Crewe, 2011a, p. 523). Extending the thoughts of Franke (1995), who noted that individuals have to comply with the wish, the desires of power, soft power and self-regulation are thus ring-fenced by a coercive nature because the full weight of the walls of hard power is looming in the background when softer responsibilising techniques fail.

When considering state responsibilisation techniques, inducement is one whereby incentives are offered to the public to undertake practices, such as in the crime control realm. This can be extended to the open prison and peer-led induction. In fact, a recent blog by the prisons inspectorate referred to the 'power of an incentivising culture' (HMCIP, 2025). The incentive in the case of induction is that by undertaking the intervention, you will have the information and tools to navigate prison life and access elevated levels of freedom and autonomy such as ROTL. If you try to opt out, you are deemed as not having the foundational skills and knowledge to navigate this stage of your sentence. As Hannah-Moffat (2000, p. 524) observes, 'an unwillingness to participate in an institutionally defined regime of empowerment can result in nothing other than punishment'. In this sense, empowerment 'is used to justify, rationalize and legitimate a variety of disciplinary techniques through as parallel discourse of responsibility' (Hannah-Moffat, 2000, p. 524).

Like many strategies within the open prison institution, peer-led induction mobilises good power in the constructed technologies of the self through participation, responsibility and empowerment. Yet, they also co-exist with enactments of power such as coercion and surveillance while prioritising the prisons own objectives. There is the element here of maintaining social order. Well-adapted prisoners are a lower risk of self-harm, suicide, mental health issues and refractory 'risky' behaviours which mean that institutional safety, compliance, order and security are more robust. An example of this is that attending induction is a voluntary endeavour; however, failing to attend or not engage appropriately results in consequences to the offender's progression and resettlement as the comment of Peter indicates.

> ...get a booklet with the timetable of induction modules [...] it's on your head to follow it and go where it says at the time it says. If

> you struggle with doing that or miss anything, then you have to wait to complete that module the next time it runs so it means that induction gets delayed which means you'll be held back moving off the induction and your progress will too. (Peter)

This combination is particularly toxic as responsibilisation coexists against a punitive backdrop that does not take in to account the experiences and circumstances of the individual prisoner and, most importantly, needs, constructing the offender as 'accountable and responsible for their actions irrespective of victimization and structural impediments' (Hannah-Moffat, 2000, p. 525). As Bosworth (2007, p. 72) argues, 'behaviour once thought to reflect socio-economic factors, psychological disturbances and/or opportunities, is in other words[. . .] a matter of choice'. Responsibilisation is subjective, and as such, individual characteristics and experiences and people's attitudes are key drivers of its success.

What is clear is the negative 'othering' of the identity of those who fail to engage or are unable to enact expectations of regulation to navigate open prison. These are the individuals in the eyes of the institution who will be unable to benefit from all the experiences and opportunities available, especially surrounding access to temporary release from the prison. Effectively, 'life becomes harder for those who do not accept responsibility for governing their own confinement' (Ballesteros-Pena, 2018, p. 459). This pressure from prison staff, also re-enforced by the induction peer support workers through the dissemination of information, acts as a technology of the self, pressuring the show of responsibility and self-regulation. The underbelly of tight forms of penal power is revealed when prisoners fail to 'subjectify themselves appropriately' (Crewe & Ievins, 2020, p. 51).

In this vein, if prisoners do not want to or are not able to functionally responsibilise themselves in the manner expected by the prison, namely 'if they choose not to conform to institutional demands, or if they cannot recognize their "best interests", then punishment and constraint are not far away' (Crewe, 2011a, p. 523). As such, ROTL being delayed, withdrawn or the return to closed conditions and higher levels of security are the broad range of methodologies of choice for punitive intervention in open conditions, or they have to remain on the induction programme longer and their progression delayed, as described by James below:

> . . .OMU [Offender Management Unit] don't come to you [. . .] it's your responsibility to contact them and find out what you need to do and submit the forms otherwise your progression and going out will be delayed.

Interestingly, while prisoners are seen as active participants in their environment under the guise of responsibilisation, the information that is shared and disseminated actually reveals that prisoners are not really steeped in the supposition that prisons can and will act freely (Bosworth, 2007). The negative consequences of failing to responsibilise themselves is shared by both staff and peers as many ex-prisoner interviewees shared:

> I got told not to do this and that [...] silly things like stepping on the grass in a certain area would mean I get sent back to closed conditions [...] the peer mentor told me that. (Harvey)

This can be situated within the observations of Bosworth (2007, p. 74) who argues that 'the true might of the prison's rigorous and punitive moral economy becomes apparent' when responsibilisation fails. To Shamir (2008, pp. 7–8) responsibilisation:

> ...assumes a moral agency which is congruent with the attributed tendencies of economic-rational actors: autonomous, self-determined and self-sustaining subjects [...] as the choice of expression for action is, or so the neo-liberal notion of rationality would have it, the expression of free will on the basis of a self-determined decision, the consequences of the action are borne by the subject alone, who is solely responsible for them.

However, it is difficult for the prisoner to be responsible for actions that lead to consequences when they are not provided with a needs-driven commensurate foundation to be autonomous or autonomous effectively. The argument is that the responsibility in the first instance lies with the responsibilising institution to provide this foundation. In this sense, it evidences what Crewe and Ievins (2020, p. 62) describe as the prison being 'inconsistent, deficient or bureaucratically lax in providing the means that would allow prisoners to become what it necessitates them to be'. Power in this sense is tight and loose, taut and slack (Crewe & Ievins, 2020), with prisoners being hammered as a square peg into a round hole without the tools to help them inhabit it correctly. There is also the notion of deficiency underpinning frustration characterised by the lack of prison engagement with the prisoners while the culture of indifference permeated interaction.

As such, there exists the indication that the prison demonstrates and operationalised form of 'authoritarian governmentality' (Dean, 1999) or 'neo-paternalism' (Crewe, 2009). I, however, deem the term 'Coercive Responsibilisation' as a more apt concept to encapsulate the responsibilising of offenders as shaping prisoner adaptation, culture and prisoner social life in distinctive ways. This builds upon the theorisation of Foucault (1977), expanded by Crewe (2011a, p. 515), identifying that power is 'diffuse and decentralised, operating in a manner that is "light" but anonymous, demanding without seeming coercive, everywhere but nowhere'. This can be further situated within the theorisation of Rose (2000, p. 333) who describes control workers as having 'a new administrative function – the administration or marginalia [...] through the identification of the riskiness of individuals, actions, forms of life and territories'.

To Ericson and Haggerty (1997, p. 41) control is 'about the generation of knowledge that allows selection of thresholds that define acceptable risks and generates practices of inclusion and exclusion based upon that knowledge'. Prisoners' fear is based upon the power of these control workers; in the open prison, the 'pen is mightier than the sword' and feeds into the insecurity and anxiety and overall fear experienced by prisoners. In this sense, the reconfigured penal power can be exemplified through officers now being able to 'mediate the forms of psychological power that are among the main sources of hope and frustration for prisoners'. They are effectively the gatekeepers, governing from a distance. While some show evidence of staff–prisoner relations improving in the face of regulation of staff power and softening of abrasive staff cultures showing potential that the adversarial divide between both parties is now bridgeable, the nature of power still has a grip on those subjected to it (Crewe, 2011a, 2011b). The inappropriate use of soft power is tantamount to an abuse of power. Although a departure from physical punishment in brutal, degrading and overt ways, soft power is just as impactful in its consequences.

The peer support function of welcoming, addressing prisoner concerns and describing their early days in custody was sorely lacking. The PSI governing induction states that 'Prisoners with wide custodial experience are likely to need less input than those comparatively new to prison, but staff should be aware that some prisoners may not retain information for very long and will need reminding' (NOMS, 2015, p. 8). However, the provision of information to those with custodial experience was seemingly reduced to a state of absence as expressed by Steve:

> Just cos I've been around the block [different prisons] don't mean I know it all or should be expected to [...] each prison is different, but they just expected me to know it and get on with it.

This also seems to neglect both the presence of the pains of *entry shock* and *adaptation* alongside a core aim of peers in the induction process who should be offering reassurance to those who arrive at the establishment. There exists a dangerous assumption that those who have been in previous establishments will have by default the requisite knowledge and skills to navigate the custodial environment. This neglects the many individual and personal factors that interact between the process of transfer and transition and the well-being of those experiences these processes. This neglects a needs-driven approach to the intervention through failure to establish each individual prisoner's circumstances.

The Peer Support Paradox

All of the ex-prisoners who were interviewed stated that they had received some form of peer support, but it is important to note that the majority of them noted that they did not receive this support through the 'official channels' of the Induction Peer Support Workers or the Induction Prison Officers. Rather, they achieved this through informal networks of friendships and allegiances that had been formed over the course of their time in the prison system.

> Luckily, I knew a few guys from some previous prisons, and they got me up to speed and helped me with what I needed to do [...] no-one else did. (Pauley)

This shows that peer support helps with the induction process but not in the way that it was intended and instead comes from peers outside of the programme. Offenders were compelled to migrate away from the peer element of that intervention that should have helped them adapt and take on a form of self-responsibility that both manifested as a fact-finding mission that shouldn't have been required. This forced them to leave a programme that should have supported and developed them as well as their knowledge of the establishment due to the deficient nature of the many factors that undermine the 'peer' function of the peer-led induction while also serving to diminish the intervention as a whole. It has led to a peer-led induction that is characterised by the absence of engagement by peers. They may well be those in the know but they are remiss to engage with mentees to exchange this information. When considering an interactionist perspective in relation to prison adjustment, it provides the foundation for a greater propensity for adjustment problems, given the imbalance between the prisoners and peers and also the prisoners and the environment. As Adams (1992, p. 281) suggests, some environments feature safety and support which is a key cornerstone of peer-led induction, with the mix of people associating being a critical feature of the environment. When that is a mismatch, adjustment will be diminished. It therefore begs the question as to why peers are needed in a formal capacity, especially as the induction is largely reduced to a didactive endeavour.

Responsibilisation in the experience of those ex-prisoners interviewed suggested that it left them in a state of ontological uncertainty (Giddens, 1984) through tying them into their own subjection. These applications of penal power create significant insecurities, and when in the face of uncertainty, offenders perceive everything as loaded with meaning and viewed through the eye of the beholder as a test or a threat. Crewe (2011a) identifies prisoners talking about being 'set up to fail'. I also heard many similar comments throughout the interviews, with the prison presented as an institution that obstructs one's progress despite attempting to create the illusion or image of seeking to help. The widespread comments from participants about 'hoops to jump through' (Paul) and 'obstacles put in our way' (Rich) are indicative of 'an encounter that is one-sided, almost designed to trip you up' (Crewe, 2011a, p. 514). Here, this ties in with the theorisation that prisoners are unsupported in doing what the institution expects and are also 'impeded and abandoned' by the institution in their efforts to do what is expected. Effectively, they are unable to meet the standards by which they are assessed and judged by for progression. This tight and loose, taut and slack construct operates in a hybrid form with a 'low demand, low assistance' conceptualisation. In this sense, 'prisoners are abandoned and invisible at least with regard to any meaningful effort [...] to help them change themselves' (Crewe & Ievins, 2020). Responsibilisation has shifted the purpose of the prison. The prison now provides the warehouse for prisoners within which the prisoners make the decisions surrounding their future. The responsibilised prisoner in the eyes of the

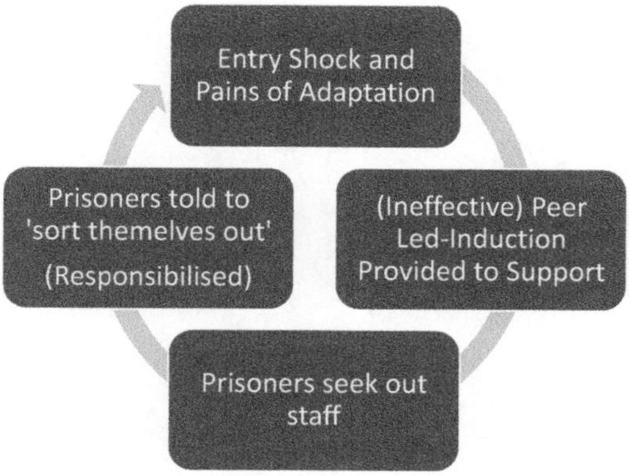

Fig. 2. Cycle of Induction Based Suffering.

institution is arguably the 'proto customer, always assessing his options. and then selecting, rationally and soberly, the best among them' (Bosworth, 2007, p. 72).

Prisoners are stuck in a devastating cycle (Fig. 2) as peer-led induction is an example of a failed policy through failure to properly design, implement and deliver the intervention. This shows a lack of commitment to it and prisoner needs, either because of a disregard for prisoner safety and well-being or for self-serving motivations that exist behind a veil of responsibilisation. As such, this, alongside the expectation of prisoners responsibilising themselves, potentially causes even more damage to a prisoner's already fragile existence through expounding the tightness associated with imprisonment, especially when considering the pains associated with prison transfer, entry and adaptation/adjustment. This serves to undermine the whole ethos behind the intervention, destabilising any notion of the intervention being perceived as legitimate or contributing to the legitimacy of the induction and prison regime.

Returning to the opening of this chapter and the ideology and expectation that peer supporters and staff should be giving their time, knowledge and support, the exploration of this notion against the backdrop of purported responsibilisation also illustrates the alarming deficiencies in the realm of information sharing and knowledge management, which were explored in the previous chapter. The book now moves on to re-conceptualise the issues and manifestations covered thus far to both consider them and their foundations and situate them within a framework of iatrogenic intervention outcomes.

Chapter 7

The Unintended Outcomes of Well-Meaning Intervention? The Iatrogenic Outcomes of Peer Support

> It is a lot better to walk alone than with a crowd going in the wrong direction. (Siu, n.d.)

The peer support model of induction has not had evaluation since a small-scale impact evaluation of a pilot study almost 20 years ago (HMPS: Safer Custody Group, 2005). In the absence of regular evaluation and in the context of the ever-changing penal landscape since, there is a lack of evidence to support that the intervention is indeed meeting its aims and objectives and delivering the intended outcomes. To reiterate, these are to: offer information and reassurance upon arrival at the institution, provide positive information and immediate reassurance, provide new arrivals with key information that will be useful to them in their early days in custody and follow up with individuals, especially those who are vulnerable or who experience difficulties that can increase their vulnerability (HMPS: Safe Custody Group, 2005). The evidence that this book offers, however, imparts that there are a range of unintended iatrogenic outcomes associated with the intervention rather than its intended ones.

This chapter aims to introduce and consider these unintended 'iatrogenic outcomes' of the peer-led induction model and the foundations for them. It does so by re-conceptualising and situating them within a framework of intervention iatrogenesis and places the intervention among the collective of '[i]nterventions that purport to modify behaviour…. [and] have the power to bring about unintended, harmful consequences' (Rhule, 2005, p. 621). Central to this is power. This consideration of how power infuses the peer-led induction illustrates the ways and extent to which this power-sharing initiative underpins and exacerbates the tightness experienced in imprisonment in greater depth, through consideration of the way that power is applied institutionally by management, induction prison staff and peer support workers. In doing so, this chapter explores the idea that peer-led induction is harmful in terms of mental health outcomes for those

Navigating Mental Health in the Male Open Prison, 127–143

doi:10.1108/978-1-83549-706-720251007

prisoners engaged with it rather than helpful. The chapter firstly establishes the pivotal concept of iatrogenesis, connecting the theorisation of Illich (1975, 1976) and Cohen (1988, 1998) within a framework of how the penal institution establishes and exacerbates the unintentional and detrimental outcomes stemming from peer-led induction. It illustrates the influence of enduring penal issues that have been charted earlier in the book and initially highlights the role of belligerence in penal policy, especially in relation to focus on actioning change and a lack of stable grounding to the peer support intervention.

It then expands this further through the conceptualisation of this as 'Institutional Pain Delivery'. It so illustrates this by situating notions of 'feathering the nest' and the 'peer support paradox', which have emerged from the findings within the context of 'managerial, staff and mentor motivations' as an abuse and misuse of power. The chapter then considers the saturation of interventions in custodial settings, connecting it to penal belligerence and establishes this through the exploration of the basis for the explosion of penal peer intervention and 'intervention-itis'. Given the observation that managerialism now dominates contemporary organisations, including a shift to pronounced hierarchical structures that 'attempt to monitor [...] through target-setting and the use of information technology' (Bennett, 2016, p. 7), it goes on to then consider how this inflammation has underpinned unintended outcomes from the intervention through the lens of 'Managerialism'. It then proceeds to establish how these areas interact and contribute to the 'Tightness of Imprisonment' that is experienced by those subjected to peer-led induction. It also considers how this tightness is experienced, by prison staff involved in the delivery of the intervention, as institutional top-down demands of managerialism influence their role.

The chapter draws to a close by reconciling the notion of iatrogenic harm emanating from the peer-led induction with that of a lack of an informed theoretical and evaluative grounding. This makes it clear that when designing, implementing and delivering prison interventions, 'in the absence of sound theory, programs stand little chance to bring about good and may even cause harm' (Welsh & Rocque, 2014, p. 262). In doing so, the chapter introduces the notion of 'Programme Theory', which is the overarching theory or model of how an intervention is expected to work (Funnell & Rogers, 2011). The culmination of these findings indicates clearly either a lack or, at the very least, severe deficiencies in the Programme Theory of the peer-led induction model, especially in terms of evaluation and the use of evaluation. This in turn creates, develops and exacerbates the harm experienced, undermining the intended outcomes of the intervention and giving rise to the host of unintended harms presented.

The Unintended Outcomes of 'Well-Meaning' Intervention

There is often a focus on the benefits and positive outcomes that can emanate from interventions put in place to help those subjected to them. In the case of induction peer support interventions, the intent is clear.

> Effective peer support can contribute to suicide prevention in the widest sense by helping to create a safe, decent, and healthy environment with positive prisoner/prisoner and staff/prisoner relationships, where prisoners' problems can be voiced and addressed. (HMP Safer Custody Group, 2005)

In relation to the actual outcomes, the previous limited evaluation of what was then a pilot scheme over 20 years ago, using a small sample comprising of 55 prisoners, 17 officers and 18 insiders across a total of 6 prisons and focused on those with limited prison experience boldly concluded that:

> The Insiders scheme has had a positive impact on prisoners' early experience of custody being both informative and reassuring. The scheme successfully adapted to suit establishments with differing functions, facilities, and populations. Those where the Insiders had been fully integrated into the everyday procedures tended to operate more smoothly. (HMPS: Safe Custody Group, 2005)

However, this appears to be a rather facile and misguided perspective when considering the deleterious intervention outcomes evidenced by this study. There is limited attention given to issues identified during the evaluation of the Insiders Scheme. In terms of the issues that were raised regarding setting up, developing and running the scheme; they only considered the voices of insiders, Prison Officers and Suicide Prevention Co-ordinators. There is far more focus on the positives, and as such, McCord (2003, pp. 27–28) perhaps sums this up best in stating that:

> Researchers typically fail to consider whether social programs have adverse effects, looking only for favourable results [...] Yet providers of social services do not have a right to harm their clients. Nor do most providers wish to do so. But the social climate that buries evidence of harm is powerful.

As Scott (2016, p. 108) suggests, total institutions, like the asylum, damage mental health rather than providing places of sanctuary or healing. As such, when considering the total institution of the prison, it can be argued that interventions, no matter how well-meaning they may be in their intent, may well be flawed by virtue of the institutional construct they are contained within. These manifest, as the book indicates, in iatrogenic harms, the 'injury, hurt or damage generated by an institutional practice which is justified on the basis of helping, assisting or healing individuals with problems requiring remedy' (Scott, 2016, p. 107).

Origins of Iatrogenesis

Emanating from a medical foundation, iatrogenesis, derived from the Greek 'iatros' (physician) and 'genesis' (origin), was a concept introduced by radical social critic Ivan Illich (1975, 1976). Its simple premise was that it conceptualised the detrimental impacts of modern medicine on society and specifically based on the manifestation of counterproductivity from medical intervention.

Illich's work, however, was not confined to just the field of medicine and was clearly applicable to a range of others with the institution being the central structure, whether that be schools creating ignorance, hospitals creating ill-health or asylums creating madness (Scott, 2016). The findings drawn upon have demonstrated support for the idea that when considering penal institutions, they create and exacerbate pain. Cohen (1988, 1998) extended the work of Illich to a criminological context. However, it is his notion of clinical iatrogenesis, which is especially relevant, can be extended to term it as prison iatrogenesis. Cohen sets out a typology of this phenomenon.

Clinical iatrogenesis is where hospitals, doctors and modes of treatment are 'themselves the sickening agents' by prescribing drugs with harmful side effects, carrying out unnecessary surgery and otherwise inflicting pain on patients (Cohen, 1988: cited in Bowling, 2011, p. 5). In a criminological setting, criminal justice actors can also cause suffering, harm and occasionally even death, aid in stigmatisation and labelling, and foster and institutionalise deviance.

In the criminological construct, Cohen viewed criminal justice agents as those who can inflict pain, injury and death with Bowling (2011, p. 5) illustrating this as 'damaging families, blighting careers, contribute to labelling and Stigmatization whilst creating and entrenching deviance within individuals'. Cohen (1988, 1998) described this as 'paradoxical damage'.

Earlier in this book, the enduring and worsening issues associated with imprisonment were illustrated and charted chronologically, utilising investigative reports into prison conditions. They are indicative not only of crime control institutions repeatedly failing to achieve their goals but also is illustrative of what Bowling (2011, p. 4) highlights the 'problem is not merely that criminal justice fails to work, in some instances it makes things worse'. As Officer Emily says in the context of peer-led induction and the goal of promoting safer custody:

> Everyone starts with best intentions to be hot [on self-harm] but then you see the attitude change [. . .] [it's] a knock-on effect from existing issues and negative staff culture.

This notion of things being made worse can be firmly situated within a criminological conceptualisation and framework of iatrogenesis. Just as Cohen (1998, p. 194) warns that no one 'aware of the history of crime control can continue advocating "more of the same" in good faith', this warning transcends into consideration of the penal estate and its design and use of interventions and programmes. As such, *paradoxical damage* and iatrogenesis provide 'an informed basis for scepticism towards benign transfer' (Cohen, 1998, p. 193), in this case being the continued expansion of penal intervention and programmes which are devoid of a meaningful foundation of theory in the design, implementation and evaluation phases and are rather based on what appears to be quite tedious and fragile notions of intent and the hope of replicating outcomes shown in other interventions and programmes. This is especially noticeable in peer support interventions, with the concept of peer support being applied in various guises without a suitable foundation to deliver the intended outcomes as evidenced in the specific construct of peer-led induction. As such, a transfer of intent to deliver positive outcomes associated with peer support transforms from an initially benign transfer to one that is potently malignant given the unintended outcomes that it produces and exacerbates.

Just as Illich (1975, 1976) viewed societal dependence of professionally based health care as a threat to health, this chapter extends that notion into the criminological landscape and the penal estate by in a similar vein conceptualising the penal institution's reliance on interventions as a threat to prisoners' well-being and health. Furthermore, just as Illich (1975, 1976) also questioned the effectiveness of the medical establishment through constructing the narrative argument that more harm than good is caused by medicine, in a penological context, this book's central narrative argues that prison intervention, both broadly and specifically in the form of peer-led induction, is illustrative of causing, reinforcing and exacerbating 'Prison Made Pain', which this chapter next considers.

The Foundations of Iatrogenic 'Prison Made Pain'

The evidence presented in this book thus far demonstrates that there are a range of negative outcomes associated with the peer-led induction intervention. This evidence demonstrates that it is delivering paradoxical and contradictory outcomes to those it is intended to deliver. A central theme arising from the data and providing the foundation for these outcomes are that they primarily stem from the motivations of management, prison staff and mentors, with these motivational factors manifesting as both abuse and misuse of power. This misuse of power involves the incorrect, careless of dishonest use of it, while abuse of power plays out as the misuse of authority to take actions in personal interest, in this case negatively impacting; the intervention, those subjected to it, those staff in the delivery of it and the institution. This is explored and illustrated through the notions of *motivation*, *feathering the nest*, the *peer support paradox* and *managerialism*.

Motivation: The Abuse and Misuse of Power

The reconfiguration of penal power in the construct of peer support as a peer-led induction endeavour sees a shift in the way power is enacted in prison. Moving away from the historic conceptualisations of power that are normally aligned with applications of power in prisons, there is the argument that good power utilised with the intent to produce the positive quality of life, safety and other custodial outcomes through power-sharing initiatives, such as the use of peer-led support in custodial settings, can achieve positive outcomes. Matthews (2014, p. 43) recognised the infusion of power in the mechanisms of the criminal justice system. From the interpersonal to the structural, power operates at every level and further considerations identify the capacity of those applying power to produce intended and foreseen effects on others; however, it is the unintended and unforeseen outcomes of reconfigured power, often neglected, to which this section now turns.

'Feathering the Nest'

Paramount to any prison is security, with it being central to debates around care and control in custodial settings. The open prison, which is the lowest security Category D rating, also has its own category-specific caveats. The Ministry of Justice states:

> The main purpose of open conditions is to assess prisoners in conditions more similar to those that they will face in the community. Time spent in open prisons affords prisoners the opportunity to find work, re-establish family ties, reintegrate into the community and ensure housing needs are met. (Prison Guide, 2022)

This is facilitated through the Release on Temporary License (ROTL) Scheme, by helping to prepare them for resettlement in the community once they are released.

When considering the motivations of prisoners for being peer support workers, a general consensus from the mentees is that the engagement of the mentors was not for altruistic reasons and was far detached from this with one interviewee describing them as:

> They are manipulators [...] out for themselves. (Joey)

Both the ex-prisoner and staff interviewees highlighted some ways that this plays out in practice. When prisoners arrive at the prison, they are not in a position to be released on ROTL straight away, and there is a period of risk assessment and consideration of the individual's specific case before ROTL can be considered. This therefore limits the movement of the newly received prisoners into the establishment. Whilst they have the freedom to leave their cells mostly freely, with the exception of observing periods in their cells during roll calls and at night-time, they are not able to leave the prison on ROTL. The freedom of other prisoners to engage with ROTL allows them the opportunity to access contraband and smuggle it into the prison or facilitate this through those in position of trust. For those working in induction, there is the opportunity for them to access a 'captive audience' with new inductees.

> They were the people supplying the drugs to people when they came in [...] first thing they asked was if I needed anything and they didn't mean support or help to get settled in. (Joey)

John described how he was targeted in the reception area when he arrived and given a 'sales pitch' that the induction insider was the person to see. Other interviewees highlighted the privileged access that the Induction prisoners had.

> They had access to all areas in the prison [...] reception, OMU, other areas of the prison that most of us can't go to. (Danny)

This access was important in many ways. As John concurred:

> They had all the power. They could access the reception area and get prop (their personal property held in storage in reception) and orders while we had to wait.

This meant, by virtue of their role, that the induction peer supporters were in a position to engage with staff in order to get catalogue orders and property which often other prisoners had to wait until a certain allocated time and date slot to receive. This often occurred when collecting prisoners from the reception areas or running 'reception and induction' related errands to this area of the prison or through the invention of fictitious reasons for attending the desired area.

> It was a pisstake. They were only in the job so that they could fly about and do their dodgy dealing and get what they wanted. (Joey)

The most contentious issue stemmed from the access these peers had to the Offender Management Unit (OMU) and staff. This is the unit that contains the staff involved in the risk assessment and ROTL issuing process. There was the perception that they were able to circumvent the normal channels of procedure to do so and oil the wheels of progressing ROTL applications and queries for themselves. This was something that was both recognised and normalised by staff, viewed as a benefit of the role among the majority of staff interviewed.

> At the end of the day they help us out dealing with the prisoners, so we do our bit for them. Last thing we need is a bunch of pissed off mentors on our case and not doing the job right.... if we keep them happy things go according to plan. (Officer Kev)

Ex-prisoner mentees had a cynical view of this involvement with OMU, with some going as far as labelling those peer support workers as 'Screw-boys' and 'Grasses'.

> They are up there in those offices snitching [...] they'd do anything to look good to the screws. (Gary)

> Who knows what info they are giving the screws [...] they're giving them something- that's why they get looked after. (Graeme)

A key issue was a lack of perceived interest in the role, which is further considered. While the Prison Service Instruction (NOMS, 2015) governing induction states that the expectation is that support be provided by Induction Insiders, there were alarming deficiencies in this area.

> They [peers] were only interested in fucking my off out the door so they could get on with cooking their dinner and association [...] questions just went unanswered- they were invisible. (Joey)

> As soon as I signed off the paperwork they needed, they were off, and that was the last time I even saw them. (James)

The comments above clearly indicate a distinct lack of interest from the peers in assisting with this process, and there was a prevalent perspective that the peers were only interested in having their paperwork signed off which indicates to others that they had 'done their job'. Ex-prisoner interviewees all agreed that the peers were using their role as a way to look good and curry favour in the eyes of the prison staff. This exposes the attempt of mentors to cultivate a superficial image to draw staff attention to the supposed altruistic nature of their role as opposed to some of the sinister underbelly, which has been outlined. Being a peer mentor/support worker in the eyes of the ex-prisoner sample is a means to an end, a self-serving motivation, a cynical move with their role the sidecar to the vehicle getting them what they want. They have power, which they apply for their own self-serving motivations which re-enforces hierarchy, but due to this, they are also viewed as Steve articulates as 'another set of screws on us and getting busy but just not in uniform'.

This, however, is just one perspective. One of the limitations of the study is that the voice of the mentors is absent due to the changes made to the study. As such, it is difficult to generalise the observations around peer support workers to all who do the job. However, the perspective of those subjected to peer-led induction is that one of the inherent and inevitable failings of the peer-led induction is quite simply that power is not always shared or applied through power-sharing as intended and that abuse of this power in a penal context is arguably inevitable.

'The Peer Support Paradox'

> Luckily, I knew a few fellas from my last prison, and they showed me the ropes and what I needed to do [...] no-one else did. (Rich)

Another prevalent manifestation of how the questionable motivations of staff and peer support workers used their power is that of the *peer support paradox*. This chapter has conceptualised these issues along with the tensions of responsibilisation, which the previous chapter has looked at extensively. It is this combination that feeds the paradox that exists.

While all of those ex-prisoner interviewees interviewed reported some level of peer support, it is essential to state here that the majority noted that they gained this support not through the 'official channels' of the induction peer support workers nor the induction prison officers but rather from informal networks of friendships and allegiances built up longitudinally through their time spent in the prison system.

This suggests that peer support works in assisting the induction process however not in an intended manner and in fact is garnered from peers outside of the programme. Offenders in this sense were forced to migrate away from a programme that should support and develop both them and their knowledge of the establishment to help them adapt and undertake a form of self-responsibilisation that both manifested as a fact-finding mission that should not have been necessary. This characterises the iatrogenic nature and outcome of intervention as the peer-led induction undermines its own premise of a structured and targeted social support programme through driving people away from peers to informal networks. Here the almost perverse notion of responsibilisation is at its most acute. Prisoners and staff involved in power-sharing results in a blurring of boundaries for prisoners while giving power to some inmates with questionable motivations causes prisoners to 'steer clear' of those who should be helping them.

Managerialism: Intervention-itis and Tick-Box Cultures

This chapter has primarily considered the motivations of induction staff and peers that underpin iatrogenic outcomes. However, it is now appropriate acknowledge the managerialist notions behind broadly, the use of peer support interventions and more specifically peer-led induction which is synonymous with 'intervention-itis'.

It also considers the impact that *managerialism* has in practice, with the top-down management negatively impacting peer-led induction and its staff ability to deliver its intended aims. This managerialism was an approach that was associated from within the public service as the vehicle to improved efficiency and effectiveness. This all too familiar trend within the public sector is often referred to as 'new public management' (Bennett, 2016; Pollitt, 1993). In the penal estate, processes of management monitoring and control were embraced as the solution to the established problems experienced in prisons such as including improving security (Learmont, 1995; Spurr & Bennett, 2008) and 'increasing management control and direction, turning good intentions into reality' (Bennett, 2016, p. 7). However, as this chapter indicates, in the case of peer-led induction, good intentions lead to an unintended reality.

'Intervention-itis'

While the chapter has introduced the perceived role motivations of the peer supporters, the gaze now turns to management and staff. It is not just the prison mentors that *feather the nest* but both management and staff are guilty of doing the same albeit in a quite different guise for the most part.

As established in the earlier chapters, there is a saturation of interventions in prison, whether its peer support or offending behaviour. The suffix 'itis' is employed as a primarily medical suffix, derived from the Greek language, used to denote inflammation. For example, appendicitis translates as the literal or figurative inflammation of the appendix. Applied to the penal context and the use of various interventions and programs with prisoners, it conceptualises this explosion of peer support through what I term as 'intervention-itis', meaning the inflamed number and usage of such interventions and programs across the penal estate, of which peer-led induction is one (Stevens et al., 2025). It illustrates the tendency of policymakers to treat enduring, systemically generated problems with limited interventions that are insufficient or inappropriate for the intended improvement. This is a problematic feature of criminal justice policy making, in England and Wales at least. It is not a new problem.

This 'itis' exists and has been expanded for a variety of reasons. From an institutional perspective surrounding peer support and peer-led induction, it has been seen by many managers as an opportunity to do more with less in the face of the growing violence of austerity within the penal estate with under-staffed and under-resourced institutions a norm in contemporary prisons across in England and Wales (Fletcher & Batty, 2012).This is symbolic of the re-configuration of power, which has seen the use of prisoners more involved in custodial provisions as such, intervention-itis is arguably a product of this clamour to paper over the cracks. All prison staff interviewed concurred staunchly with this assessment whether it being a primary of secondary aim.

> It makes sense from the higher ups [. . .] saves them resources and plugs the gaps that exist [. . .] I guess its clever management or maybe desperation. (Officer Lily)

> They just trot things out willy-nilly, without any though about the logistics and practicality [. . .] they just want a quick fix, no thought about how to go about it though. (Officer Kev)

Also, this view was similarly held by a considerable number of ex-prisoner interviewees. Interviewees from the ex-prisoner sample were firmly of the belief that the use of peer supporters in the intervention was a ploy to plug the gaps arising from a lack of resources in personnel in the penal establishments.

> All they are trying to do is put the dairy [responsibility] on us [. . .] they ain't got the staff to do what they are meant to do so they've got the screw boys running about doing their job for them. (Chris)

> We have to rely on the peer supporters to do a lot of what we should do – making sure they have a phone call, answering concerns and queries, reassuring them [. . .] the peers are there to supplement us not replace us and do our duties for us. (Officer Kev)

> I wouldn't tell them this, but they are a god send for me personally [...] we haven't got the bodies on the landings anymore to even do the basics [...] they free us up. (Officer Emily)

In this sense, the staff recognised the influence of peers on their workload. This is something that they believed management had also realised, and this is situated firmly within the framework of Boyce et al. (2009, p. 12), who recognise using peers to reduce workload 'sold it to the prison', especially as it is evidenced that peers ease professional pressure, extend support and reduce staff turnover as well as being cost-effective (Boyce et al., 2009; Fletcher & Batty, 2012). This is an initial illustration of a managerialist approach to the use of peer support, 'weaponising' it as a tool to facilitate their self-serving cultures of institutional compliance.

As Bennett (2016, p. 8) muses, '[p]risons in England and Wales have seen the proliferation of the technologies and techniques of target-setting and monitoring in a quite pronounced form over the last 25 years. This has included the introduction of key performance targets (KPTs) and indicators, audits, and ratings systems'. The use of peer support interventions, and specifically peer-led induction, is symbolic of a top-down approach with the strategic direction, policy and planning devised by prison management. From these strategic plans, management develops the policies and action plans required to meet the strategic goals and passes them on down to the boots on the floor to implement.

This top-down approach is viewed among the staff interviewees as very exclusionary, as it precludes staff involvement in developing its policies, plans and directions from their ideas, suggestions and solutions and as such reduces the ability for employee participation in decision-making, problem-solving and strategic planning. The staff cited this as one of the key reasons for a lack of interest and job dissatisfaction.

> I've been in the job too long now to bother trying to talk to them [management], they ain't interested in what we've got to say [...]. (Officer Woody)
>
> There was also a sense of frustration amongst the staff interviewees, with many feeling disempowered by their lack of input into policy and intervention design and implementation.
>
> If they bothered to ask us or listened when we tried to feedback and acted upon it [...] things would be so much better. (Officer Emily)
>
> I mean, we are the ones doing this day in and day out [...] we see where the issues lie, what they are [...] it's not a quick fix admittedly but it can be improved [induction]. (Officer Kev)

Prison staff are 'agents of power' (Spierenburg, 2000), and as such, any instance of power being exercised is an opportunity to gain knowledge and provide feedback to other agents of power about the implementation of commands, policies and procedures. In this sense, as Foucault (1977) argues, it has productive and integrative impacts rather than being associated routinely as just repressive. Resonating with the ideas surrounding power, Elias (1984) states that power is two sided, operating from the top down as well as the bottom-up. However, the bottom-up approach is largely untapped, and the distribution of power is unequal. Management may be more powerful than prison staff at junior levels; however, that does not mean that they are left without power completely. This also invariably and profoundly feeds into literature surrounding the notions of a failure to design and evaluate interventions properly, from a bottom-up approach, in the rush to push programmes into practice and implement them. There have already been a number of high-profile interventions in penal settings, especially in the offending behaviour/rehabilitation realm that have been shown to be ineffective due to a lack of evidence base and evaluation (Shaw, 2019). Yet, in the clamour to paper over the cracks, issues among and within intervention are neglected. As such, the plentiful interventions bypass a number of key steps and jump the implementation phase and lack appropriate consideration of the design and construction of the intervention. This leaves the prison system in a state of intervention-itis with a plethora of interventions, such as peer-led induction, due to deficiencies in design and operation stemming from a managerialist approach to plug gaps in their institutions, which do not deliver their aims. This intervention-itis is, therefore, firmly a pre-cursor to, and source of, the iatrogenic harm established.

The persistence of ineffective interventions in prison settings can also be understood through the lens of pathway dependency, which constrains institutional decision-making, making it difficult to abandon entrenched but ineffective practices (Guiney & Yeomans, 2023). Peer-led schemes are often shaped more by the procedural demands of the institution than by an organic process of prisoner-led support. This means that rather than adapting to meet the mental health needs of those incarcerated, they often reinforce pre-existing penal logics, including a managerialist emphasis on compliance, responsibilisation and cost-effectiveness rather than genuine care. The result is an iatrogenic effect where the very interventions intended to support prisoners may exacerbate distress. Path dependency sustains intervention-itis; because penal institutions resist major reforms, rather than eliminating failed interventions, they layer new ones on top. This leads to a proliferation of short-term 'fixes' rather than structural change. This notion is explored further when considering the domain of programme theory.

'Papering Over the Cracks and Ticking the Box'

The role of management is something that can be considered further through the context of its KPTs, which cover five categories: 'Decency & Health' (such as suicide and self-harm audit score, time unlocked); 'Organisational Efficiency & Effectiveness' (such as completion of staff appraisals, timely responses to prisoner complaints and public correspondence), 'Regimes' (such as purposeful activity and the attainment of qualifications by prisoners); 'Safety' (such as assaults and accidents) and 'Security' (such as escapes, breach of temporary release and completion of searches). Of particular relevance to this book and its exploration is Decency and Health. The measure of these targets has a high visibility, being discussed at all levels. They are monitored at senior management team meetings and at performance meetings. They are described as 'visible assessment of individual, team and prison performance and were constantly in the consciousness of managers' (Bennett, 2016, pp. 74–75). These arguably drive a relentless pressure on staff to deliver the targets as the boots on the floor which some interviewees expressed:

> They are relentless [. . .] the only time we see them is when they are chasing us up for not meeting a target or ticking a box [. . .] always the negatives, the things that affect them. (Officer Emily)

Here, the perceived focus of management connects firmly with literature which indicates that the primary concern of first- and middle-line managers is to ensure they are meeting targets, delivering the business plan and ensuring audit compliance (Crewe, 2007).

Given that peer-led induction is situated firmly in the Decency and Health category and a key intervention to reduce suicide and self-harm in custody, it is a prominent focus of management which filters down to staff. Staff interviewees described the pressure they feel which then draws them away from what they feel they should be doing within the context of induction:

> If I could split myself into pieces and be in more than one place at once I could do what is really needed. (Office Lily)

> Doing a first night interview and putting a comment on the prisoners P-NOMIS [the electronic custodial record for a prisoner] is the best I can do with the time I've got. (Officer Kev)

Here, the tick-box nature of managerialism in the context of peer-led induction is vivid among the staff involved in the delivery and facilitation of the peer-led induction. Performance is no longer evaluated by the meeting the specific needs of the individual prisoner and is instead based upon 'meeting measurable targets [like] [. . .] meticulous record-keeping [. . .] the management or even the control of risk' (Cheliotis, 2008, p. 247). The prisoners are reduced to statistics to be managed within an interpersonal framework.

> It's just another example of arse-covering and crossing off another thing on their action plan. (Officer Kev)

> They put something in place, tick their box then we are left to try and make it happen [. . .] Induction is no different. (Officer Woody)

These are viewpoints echoed by all of the staff interviewees. It shows peer-led induction is clearly viewed as a managerialist measure to tick their (the manager's) own box of satisfying safer custody requirements and recommendations and the KPTs that they are subjected too. All of this comes at the expense of it being a suitably resourced intervention to have intended positive outcomes. In this sense, it actually becomes a disingenuous endeavour by management and staff, unable and incapable to deliver what is needed by those coming into the prison post transfer. It is symbolic of interplay between both misuse and abuse of power, initially from management and then the knock-on effect to staff also.

What becomes clear is that the application of power still leads to negative outcomes for those subject to it irrespective of it being applied hard or soft. In this sense, the application of power is merely shifted. Power is still applied, and it causes negative outcomes; however, these become less of a spectacle, hidden or buried under the guise of being applied in 'well-meaning or well-intended' forms and constructs, such as peer-led induction. Yet, the reality is that it is still aligned with the enduring issues documented in prisons within this book and causing pain for those subjected to it.

Tightness

How power is applied and enacted alters the experience of imprisonment. Power is experienced as both firm and soft in the open prison. There are elements of oppressiveness that characterise all penal institutions, yet there is also a deftness to them, a light touch. Rather than being a suppressive force weighing prisoners down like a millstone around their neck, it acts as a straitjacket, constraining them, by wrapping them up, smothering them and egging them on to demonstrate institutional appeasing behaviours. It best 'captures the feelings of tension and anxiety generated by uncertainty' (Crewe, 2011a; Freeman & Seymour, 2010). The iatrogenic outcomes stemming from peer-led induction have been detailed and explored with their foundations established in this chapter alongside the preceding two chapters. What these findings all illustrate is the *tightness of imprisonment*.

There is the notion that responsibilising prisoners to navigate their day-to-day prison life with greater autonomy and the variety in delivery of the design and delivery of the peer-led induction actually combines to 'set prisoners up to fail' increasing their fear of uncertainty. Tightness as a concept captures those feelings, anxieties and tensions associated with uncertainty. It encapsulates the feelings demonstrated by a number of ex-prisoner interviewees in Chapter 6, who spoke of the sense of the unknown, not knowing what to do, when to do it or how to do it for fear of getting it wrong. They put themselves under their own form of disciplinary gaze born from institutional expectations of responsibilisation. The softening of penal power underpins the notion of responsibilising prisoners.

It also feeds into more contemporary pains of imprisonment such as *entry shock* and *pain of adaptation* (Jones, 2007) with some ex-prisoners stating that anxiety associated with their transfer and change of circumstances increased in the face of a lack of needs driven support in induction. As Crewe (2011a) argues, the notions of self-governance and responsibilisation combine. Here, as the majority of the formerly imprisoned sample indicated, the sense of self and the fragility of their status in this transient phase is both challenged and eroded underpinning deleterious psychological impacts. This combination actively underpins the uncertainty that is conceptualised by tightness. There are difficulties surrounding prisoners becoming self-regulators, especially in this open prison estate. The low staffing and levels of security mean that there are options for prisoners to leave of their own accord, and as Crewe and Ievins (2020) indicate, this leads to institutional regulation shifting locus to one that is left almost in its entirety to the prisoner themselves. When support was most needed from mentors and staff, it was nowhere to be found, or when the 'physical' people were found, they hid behind a range of questionable motivations, as established in earlier chapters, to avoid engaging. This resonates with a majority of ex-prisoner interviewees who can find their frustrations situated within Crewe's (2015) theorisation of tightness whereby they spoke of difficulties navigating administration, getting answers to questions which were met with indifference and unresponsiveness. This evidences the notion of power being both 'tight and loose, taut and slack' (Crewe & Ievins, 2020). In this sense, prisoners are unsupported to become the self that is desired by the prison, and they also as a result face being impeded in their efforts to become that version of the self the institution wants them to aspire to. There is a non-optic perspective (Alford, 2000; Crewe & Ievins, 2020) where truly little is done for prisoners. They are rendered as abandoned and invisible, notions conveyed in earlier chapters, and there lacks meaningful engagement from the peer-led induction, which should be there to help them.

Managerialism in the context of induction impacts the prisoner outcomes. The staff interviewees were all of the opinion that the managerial pressure and focus on 'pen pushing' prevents them from having commensurate engagement with prisoners to facilitate and support the peer-led induction. These feed into the notion of the *peer support paradox* and makes it more malignant. Not only do prisoners migrate away from the peers that are there to supposedly support them but they also migrate away from the staff who are there to support them also due to a lack of staff availability and accessibility. This not only underpins the aforementioned pains of imprisonment but also those associated with self-regulation and governance. Prisoners in this unfamiliar environment with greater autonomy, in an open prison, with trigger points of acute mental health issues, were being left to self-regulate and navigate their sentence devoid of the support systems that are intended to alleviate the pains associated with settling into a new establishment. Prisoners are in a self-regulating environment, which is magnified in the open prison estate. In order to maintain their status in the prison and progress, they have to regulate and conform, jumping through hoops almost to satisfy those gatekeepers to freedom, with the knowledge omnipresent that if they do not, they miss out on their progression and indeed could face regression. Here, the power is waiting in the wings in a more oppressive and overt nature to act swiftly in the absence of self-regulation associated with soft application. Here, penal power is seen in its true form exerting what Crewe (2011a, 2011b) identifies as a 'grip' upon the prisoner. Bureaucracy and processes of responsibilisation combine to stifle the prisoner.

It is not just prisoners who are 'doing time' inside the prison; prison staff are also doing time and, in a number of cases, significantly longer sentences than those imprisoned by the courts. An interesting observation arising from the fieldwork was the notion that staff are subject to their own pains of imprisonment stemming from managerialism and top-down pressure, which leads to them experiencing their own form of tightness. Just like prisoners, these officers face fear, anxiety and mental duress, uncertainty, lack autonomy and face both isolation and alienation (Crewe, 2011b; Scott, 2006). These often manifest in or exacerbate pain, and Scott (2006, p. 29) captures the essence of this best in stating 'those who perform dehumanising tasks become themselves dehumanised', those who inflict pain have pain inflicted upon themselves.

> I'm always dreading what's going to happen if I can't do something or do it how they want it done [...] they sit in their meetings and behind their desks watching and monitoring hovering in the background ready to hammer us. (Officer Kev)

The staff inability to have what they deemed as adequate involvement in the peer-led induction to do the job they feel they should be doing, partly due to resourcing issues alongside the demands of meeting targets, combined to elicit fear and pressure among them, with this relentless top-down managerialism resulting in staff experiencing their own form of tightness. Tightness in this sense was a direct result of managerialism. The vice-like grip of tightness compelled the staff to feel a profound level of uncertainty. Just as ex-prisoner interviewees mirror the literature of being tied into responsibilisation and governance of the self, the same applies to the prison officers. As earlier stated in this chapter, staff expressed fear from management with them waiting to crack down on them should they not satisfy the demands handed down to them.

What is key, and a cornerstone of this book, is to illuminate the importance of not ignoring the particularly important lessons that can be garnered from interventions that fail to work or cause harm. The position of this researcher concurs with Zane et al. (2016, p. 153), who assert that 'the focus on positive results is too narrow', attributing this partly to the failure to acknowledge or even recognise that some intervention cause harm. This can lead to what they go on to describe as an 'under-appreciation of what is truly at stake in designing social interventions' (Zane et al., 2016), which is a responsibility that should be at the forefront of any programme design.

What is also relevant and apparent with the peer-led induction model is that an intervention 'not sufficiently grounded in sound [evidence and underpinned by] criminological theory is unlikely to succeed and may do more harm than good' (Zane et al., 2016, p. 153), and this connects to the much earlier notions of iatrogenesis offered by Illich (1975, 1976). As such, it is key, as Zane et al. (2016, pp. 153–154) advance, to 'determine the theoretical basis for why some programmes cause harm [...] representing an important consideration when designing future social interventions, both to diminish risk of harm and to allow for a more nuanced understanding of intervention effects'. This study has also recognised and illustrated this notion. These notions further feed into the importance of ensuring that there is an effective and evaluated Programme Theory, which is the overarching theory or model of how an intervention is expected to work. So far, the culmination of the findings has indicated either a lack or at the very least, severe deficiencies in the Programme Theory of the peer-led induction model and evaluation of it. The next chapter now considers this further.

Chapter 8

Programme Theory: Absences and Deficiencies

> It is of course possible to achieve high levels of quality and safety on the basis of intuition derived from experience alone, with little evident help from formal theory. The few successful examples that exist do not, however, help to build a science. (Davidoff et al., 2015)

Programme Theory is a tool to help people 'better understand what works, for whom and under what circumstances' (Maden et al., 2017, p. 2). The initial stage of planning an effective treatment programme involves a solid theoretical foundation on which to base the intervention (Rossi et al., 2004). This involves the foundation of a theory of programme change, which is namely how will the treatment elicit change in those subjected to it. Because of the significance of Programme Theory, advancements in evaluation literature, like logic models, have been made. These models explain how a programme functions (or is intended to function) in terms of inputs, resources, activities, outputs, outcomes and long-term impact (Mertens & Wilson, 2012). The benefits that extend from Programme Theory include a more efficient development period for interventions, optimal design and effectiveness alongside awareness of context in order to identify the best conditions for success and to enhance learning from the intervention (Davidoff et al., 2015; Zane et al., 2016).

In the context of crime prevention, theory failure has been identified as being responsible for the ineffectiveness of many penal interventions (see Scared Straight programmes-Welsh & Rocque, 2014). Given the fragility of such programmes, this author extends that proposition and its position is that the evidence supports a partial theory failure within peer-led induction as being responsible for its iatrogenic effects.

It has been documented that 'crime policy on the whole lacks a rational foundation' (Mears, 2007, p. 679), and this book has established that this could be extended to many penal interventions implemented across the estate. While there

Navigating Mental Health in the Male Open Prison, 145–153

doi:10.1108/978-1-83549-706-720251008

is a rational basis for the peer-led induction, it has been evidenced as one that is naïve and beset by a lack of consideration and context specific though in the design, implementation and delivery. Typically, policymakers and CJS management have shown a predisposition to a disproportionate focus on 'what works', but as Zane et al. (2016) proffer, 'this may ignore important lessons that can be gleaned from programmes that fail to work or even cause harm'. A second, related result is that preventative programmes without a solid theoretical foundation in criminology are unlikely to be effective and might potentially cause more harm than good. In order to reduce the risk of harm and allow for a more nuanced approach, it is crucial to understand the theoretical underpinnings of why some programmes have the potential to harm.

There seems to be the belief and premise across CJS and especially among the prison sector that peer support will work across different interventions to produce specific outcomes in differing contexts, as is the case of peer-led induction (HMPS: Safer Custody Group, 2005), because there has been some success for it in others. This, however, 'fails to recognise that some treatments cause harm' such as inability to 'cope with life' (McCord, 2003, p. 17). This is a form of generalisation that is immensely harmful to those subjected to the intervention. In the absence of an explicit account of an intervention, what staff and prisoner interviewees have described is symbolic of a manifestation to 'cargo cult science' (Feynman, 1974) whereby things that looked like science are not. More specifically, in the sphere of peer intervention, this would be 'the refusal to accept results that are "wrong" only insofar as they disagree with those obtained by an eminence' (Hanlon, 2013, p. 52). Here, the poor understanding of what the peer-led induction consists of, what it does and how it works, combine to thwart meaningful replication of the interventions that were successful. Here, that is the principle of peer support. There is a lack of engagement with the theoretical underpinnings of peer support discussed again below, and this lack of awareness and understanding of the foundations of peer support and the subtleties of it and its outcomes. This leads to an 'under-appreciation of what is truly at stake in designing social interventions' (Zane et al., 2016), a sentiment that was echoed by those interviewed who were subject to the induction interventions. In fact, literature suggests that even those that are successful are difficult to 'sustain or replicate in new contexts' (Davidoff et al., 2015).

There is some evidence of the presence of theory in the pilot review of the Induction Insider Scheme, but it is naïvely applied, extrapolating tenets of the benefits of peer support and attempting to apply them to an induction intervention without considering factors that can challenge that, as well as failing to recognise the complexity in doing so. Meaningful Programme Theory employs the combination of informal and formal theory to recognise the issue (elevated mental health issues manifesting in self-harm and suicide); identify its cause (transfer adaptation and lack of support); say what the corrective intervention is made up of (its component parts); specify the range of outcomes (desired or not); indicate why it is likely to deliver the desired results so, namely the mechanisms to do so; and describe how it will be assessed. Yes, there are guiding principles that are presented in Prison Service Instructions (PSIs) and Prison Service Orders surrounding induction. However, there is little evidence of a coherent theoretical model to bring the intended outcomes, and it does not draw or make explicit that it draws upon mainstream criminological theories (Mears, 2007). If this was given the highest standard of quality through accreditation, as Offending Behaviour Programmes are, it would need to be fully manualised, totalling five manuals (as described in Table 3).

This level of accreditation would allow for a structure to be applied to deliver the highest standards for the development, implementation and maintenance of the peer-led induction and meet the needs of those participating in it. Yet, these are reserved for Offending Behaviour Programmes.

The Buffering Model earlier discussed is completely undermined by the issues that have been presented. The theory advances that social support has a significant positive effect when individuals are under high stress and that when social support is high, individuals would develop fewer psychological problems. If peer-led induction was to utilise this theory in its programme, the induction would do as it should do; act as a buffer and maximise the ability of the individual to

Table 3. Manual Categories for Accredited Programmes.

Manual	Description
Theory manual	Details the theory and its supporting research evidence that underpins the programmes model of change
Programme manual	Details each programme session and links to the targets for change to the model of change presented in the theory manual
Assessment and evaluation manual	Provides full details, including administration, scoring and interpretation for all the measures used for assessment and evaluation within the programme
Management manual	Details the procedures for staff selection, training and appraisal; the criteria for the selection and assessment of offenders for the programme; operating conditions, procedures for monitoring and evaluating the programme and the roles and responsibilities of staff relating to the programme
Staff training manual	Provides details of all training for those staff involved in the programme, including both management and delivery personnel, alongside the procedures for assuring the competence of staff and regular reviews of staff performance

Source: Hollin and Palmer (2006, p. 14).

cope with the situation of prison adaptation. The induction does not do this, with the potential outcomes of theory application being presented as a rationale for the peer intervention, yet demonstrating no meaningful or explicit engagement with the underlying theory relating to Social Learning Theory and Differential Association Theory and lacking any understanding of how this theoretical basis interacts with the means to deliver well intended aims and objectives of the intervention. Notions of emotional support alongside being a source of practical support and other information hallmarks of a social support system are negated by the issues presented. That leaves a limited buffer effect, meaning that the prisoner is exposed to the cold front of pain emanating from entry and adaptation with little shelter. When we consider the comments from ex-prisoner interviewees, the motivations of the peer supporters interact to render the potential impact of Social Learning Theory and Differential Association Theory as a negative one; prisoners are drawn away from those peer support workers that they should be engaging experientially with and modelling. The non-altruistic nature of those delivering the peer intervention a key factor behind this. In fact, what the behaviour of the peer supporters does is to breed indifference and present a set of behaviours that are undesirable to be replicated in the open prison environment such as manipulation.

There is no explicit portrayal of theory in the evaluation of the pilot study of the Induction Insiders Scheme considering the immense variability across interventions delivering peer-led support, and this is supported by comments from officer interviewees. What exists, when considering the staff interviewees consensus, is vague and generic, lacking specificity, a contextual awareness and substance as to the how, the why and the delivery in practice. A central frustration of the staff interviewees that relates to this was the lack of thought that went into the design and implementations of peer-led induction. All too familiar, for the motivations demonstrated in this book, a prominent feature of prison interventions and true in the case of peer-led induction, is the tendency to move straight to the implementation phase. This is arguably a product of 'intervention-itis' and underpins the iatrogenic outcomes associated with the intervention.

> We use our experience and what we think is needed to pull it together. (Officer Emily)

This is a sentiment echoed throughout the prison officers interviewed. The peer-led inductions were largely experiential. While this has value, it exposes the intervention, and it exposes variability among the staff and how they carry out their role. Two of the staff interviewees in roles delivering peer-led induction had only been in service for under 4 years and had limited exposure to the prison and penal system. As such, the experience they have, although valuable, is limited, which in turn limits the scope of their experiential knowledge into intervention design and delivery. This connects also to Davidoff et al. (2015, p. 228), who recognise urgent need for more effective use of formal theory in intervention, 'because personal intuition is often biased, distorted and limited in scope' and maximum exploitation of learning and accumulation of knowledge. Promoting the transfer of learning from one project, one context and one challenge to the next is best achieved using formal theory.

One of the earlier staff comments spoke about the institution rushing out interventions without considered development using a bottom-up approach. This resonates with Davidoff et al. (2015) who identify this feature of many interventions being the tendency to move straight to implementation and circumventing the working out of the Programme Theory. The clamour to introduce the programme and keep it running has resulted in an intervention that, while being attractive superficially, lacks a clear and specific evidenced process and narrative regarding each intervention and the behavioural, social and technical processes that they seek to alter or assist.

Evaluation: Underpinning or Undermining Theory

Despite there being a clear need and rationale for programme/intervention evaluation for public sector institutions to monitor and improve performance, the reality is that very few evaluations are conducted in prisons despite an elevated level of importance for intervention in these contexts (Arseneault et al., 2016). What is important to consider in the context of peer-led induction is that it is not accredited, and so there is no obligation to ensure that it is evaluated and designed based on the best available evidence.

> I've never done anything formal. We just ask from time to time how the prisoners got on with induction and if everything is alright. They don't tend to say too much. (Officer Lily)

Of greatest relevance to this intervention is the invaluable role Programme Theory plays in providing a scaffold for evaluation. This is key because all interventions need to be designed in a manner that makes it possible and visible to ascertain whether the intervention has indeed resulted in the desired outcomes. The element of evaluation and the process of negotiation and renegotiation in the peer-led induction is absent, which means it is absent from contributing to a Programme Theory that is robust and from determining an intervention that is delivering what is intended. Here, evaluation acts as addressing whether or not 'chains of objectives' are met (Suchman, 1967, p. 55) with the Programme Theory guiding evaluation.

> I've never seen any research done on it, not since I've been here. We have a comment box, but I've not known prisoners to put feedback in there apart from complaints about more general aspects of prison. (Officer Kev)

> They never asked me what I thought about it [...] besides even if I said anything they are just going to make my life difficult and cause me a problem. (Joey)

A key challenge in designing effective peer-led interventions is escaping the constraints of pathway dependency, which described as the institutional tendency to continue along an established trajectory, even when alternative models could yield better outcomes (Guiney & Yeomans, 2023). Without a programme theory that actively challenges these entrenched patterns, reforms risk being absorbed into the wider penal logic, reinforcing institutional priorities rather than the needs of prisoners. To counteract this, a theory-driven approach must incorporate critical engagement with why past interventions have failed and ensure that new models are not merely adapted versions of previous penal policies but fundamentally reoriented towards rehabilitation, agency and structural change. The key proposition a value of Programme Theory Evaluation (PTE) is understanding why and how interventions do or do not work. The ability to evaluate the steps in a theory, as earlier mentioned, in the intervention provides an important narrative about failure and success of the differing elements in reaching its goals or aims. An inability to evaluate means there is little opportunity to not only identify what does and does not work but also why, in the context of peer-led induction, what critical mechanisms were lacking in the model, such as it being activating and engaging. This is clear evidence of the earlier consideration of Fletcher and Batty (2012), who highlighted a lack of evidence demonstrating a clear added benefit of utilising peer support, due to the lack of evaluation.

This is a theme within the MOJ, who have also failed to evaluate 20 of their accredited Offending Behaviour Programmes (Shaw, 2019). A lack of PTE also precludes the ability to identify causal attribution to determine whether the intervention caused the observed outcome and providing robust evidence of doing so. Principles of delivering and maintaining effective practice are neglected seemingly as this intervention exists outside of an Offending Behaviour framework; therefore, no evaluation or audit is attached. A core consideration of evaluation needs to be to improve the intervention, and this was lacking.

> We are the ones doing this day in and day out [...] we are able to adapt and change things about that we think need it amongst ourselves. (Officer Emily)

That is not to say there is no presence of evaluation. There appears from the data to be a type of formative assessment that takes place informally among staff. Here, any questions relating to the effectiveness of the intervention take the form of conversations between staff and handovers, as Rogers et al. (2000, p. 9) suggest, 'guiding daily actions and decisions', rather than summative considerations of effectiveness stemming from structural issues relating to the intervention. This form of functional evaluation is not to develop the Peer Led Intervention as such, but more to assist staff in the planning and management of the prison function. It sits firmly within a managerialist framework regarding motivation rather than delivering the intended aims and objectives in relation to prisoner outcomes.

Overall, the peer-led induction cannot in its construct fit within a framework of 'Effective Interventions' that the MOJ (2022) promote. These principles are documented in relation to Offending Behaviour Programmes and Interventions, yet not seemingly applied to peer-led induction. As a non-accredited programme or one that does not target Offending Behaviour, arguably it is seemingly not deemed as requiring such rigour: an evidence-based rationale, being delivered as intended and evaluation. However, these are principles that should, given the flaws in this intervention, be applied to peer-led induction and indeed all interventions that involve those who are imprisoned to ensure that they run to the highest standards and deliver their intended outcomes. There is no significant adherence to principles of effective practice, and there is 'no clear theoretical model of change, fully articulated in a Theory Manual, which explains the principles by which the programme will achieve the intended outcome' (Hollin & Palmer, 2006, p. 12). Arguably in the face of this evidence, the only purpose it serves is to plug a void and tick a box rather than a robust one that genuinely attempts to deliver the best possible outcomes employing effective practice in both development, implementation and maintenance phases.

'Bad Things Happen When Good People Pretend There Is Nothing Wrong' (Taylor, 2022)

The oft-ignored possibility of iatrogenic effects of social interventions carries important implications for research, policy and practice. First, while it would be easy enough to dismiss a study with null or negative effects and simply 'move on', studying why a social intervention did not work, or even caused harm, is a critical component of connecting sound developmental theory with penal intervention (Poulin et al., 2001).

As Bowling suggests, '[t]he unintended and ironic, but also predictable consequences of intervention are well established' (2011, p. 12). Yet despite this, they often remain unchanged and even unchallenged. The same can be said of well-intended interventions, whether they be Offending Behaviour Programs to modify behaviours and reduce re-offending, or the raft of other interventions implemented and enacted in prisons to promote positive outcomes for those who are imprisoned, with this raft of intervention creating the climate of 'intervention-itis'.

Arguably, this historic lack of contestation and change is symbolic of denial, namely 'when people are presented with information that is too disturbing, threatening, or anomalous [. . .] [it] is therefore repressed, disavowed, pushed aside or re-interpreted' (Cohen, 2001, p. 1). Peer support in custodial settings as established in this book is a staple of prison intervention, with a wealth of literature lauding its virtues and positive impact. As such, challenges to its efficacy are arguable indicators that the premise for intervention, as well as the design, implementation and delivery of interventions, is potentially flawed. Guiney and Yeomans (2023) highlight the co-existing role of pathway dependency in shaping penal policies, where historical institutional structures create a self-reinforcing cycle that limits the potential for transformative reform. In the case of peer-led induction schemes, their development is often shaped by existing bureaucratic logics rather than by empirical evidence of effectiveness. This results in schemes that replicate past models even when those models fail to achieve meaningful outcomes. Without a structured framework that acknowledges and addresses the influence of institutional inertia, peer-led interventions risk becoming yet another example of penal drift, where policies continue due to established routines rather than their demonstrated impact on prisoner well-being. Therefore, the lack of programme/intervention evaluation and change is firmly situated in the enactment of managerialism alongside fear of the identification of intervention flaws and denial. If it were not, evaluation and a theory of change to ensure that the intervention was meeting its aims and intended outcomes would surely be a much more prominent feature of the penal systems priorities. Yet the lack of action and practice illustrates the polar opposite. This book and its empirical foundation forms, arguably, a foundation for a Programme Theory for peer-led induction as it contains evaluative empirical evidence that can be used through adaptation as a guideline for informing a programme theory and evaluation. What is crucial is to design interventions with a clear hybrid of Programme Theory and an Accompanying Logic Model. The use of the logic model is important. Logic models are useful for providing a clear illustrative diagram of programme theory in a manner that is accessible and understandable to a wide range of people who come into contact with it. It can take the form of guiding those facilitating and delivering the intervention and also illuminating key concepts for those concerned with its evaluation. By employing this research study, which identifies a range of unintended outcomes diminishing the intended aims and objectives of the intervention, it allows for the process of renegotiation to occur through the redesign of the programme, highlighting the importance of evaluation to indicate areas requiring this focus.

The reconfiguration of penal power has reconfigured the pain of imprisonment and its forms and application and invariably and the experience of this imprisonment. Here, the hybrid theory of Foucault and Elias introduced earlier plays out, whereby the locus of power has changed and the enactment of punishment is less visible and less of a spectacle. These changes in power have resulted in changes in the experience of imprisonment and prisoner outcomes. What also becomes clear is that the application of power still leads to negative outcomes for those subject to it, irrespective of it being applied hard or soft. In this sense, the application of power is merely shifted. Power is still applied, and it causes negative outcomes. However, these become less of a spectacle, hidden or buried under the guise of being applied in well-meaning or well-intended forms and constructs, such as prison interventions. How those involved in the implementation and delivery of intervention apply their power also impacts how it is experienced. As Crewe (2011a, pp. 512–513) suggests, the reconfiguration of penal power in prisons in England and Wales has 'worked alongside established pains in determining the experience of imprisonment, but they are different in their sources, their feel and their effects'.

The reality is that power is still aligned with the many of the enduring issues documented in prisons within this book, causing pain for those subjected to it. In the construct of peer support interventions, the combination of these elements is best conceptualised through tightness, a vice like grip on those that come into contact with it.

Chapter 9

Unintended Harm, Unresolved Challenges: Concluding Thoughts

> Most misunderstandings in the world could be avoided if people would simply take the time to ask, "What else could this mean?". (Shannon L. Alder, n.d.)

Policymakers and prison management within the penal estate have arguably seen peer support as the panacea to bridge the plethora of enduring issues documented in this book. They appear seduced by its successes in other areas and as such laud it as a success in this sphere, blinded by its virtues or blinkered to anything other than its function in papering over the systemic cracks. However, this book argues that it is a 'golden goose' that is being asphyxiated due to issues surrounding its design, implementation and delivery. Therefore, the worry of peer-led induction being a one-size-fits-all approach that actually fits nothing or nobody is realised not by it being a prescriptive uniform offering but more by its chaotic implementation and delivery. This is an implementation that is beset by structural and operational issues that render it as yet another intervention used by managerialists and policymakers as an emergency tourniquet to stem the flow of blood while the penal system inevitable continues to bleed out, devoid from long-term life-saving attention. The concept of 'intervention-itis' has been introduced; and peer support interventions, specifically peer-led induction, are arguably the product and an illustration of this and a pathway dependency where there is still institutional resistance and impediments to change despite reformatory attempts. The pain of imprisonment is profound, and the thought that peer support is the solution by virtue of it being perceived as the solution for issues surrounding mental health, self-harm and suicide in early stages of custody and other areas of deficiency in prison is synonymous with a level of arrogance and naivety in equal measure of those in policy and management. As Ismail (2020, 2022) suggest, a culture of silence and insufficient action to contest austerity have perpetuated its acceptance and implementation, challenging prisoners' access to appropriate healthcare and support while also undermining the working conditions of prison staff.

Navigating Mental Health in the Male Open Prison, 155–164

Published under exclusive licence by Emerald Publishing Limited
doi:10.1108/978-1-83549-706-720251009

In keeping with the medical theme within which the roots of the book's core conceptualisation of iatrogenesis are founded, it can be said that while peer intervention is intended to heal the wounds of the pain of imprisonment, what it in fact does is worsen the existing wound and create new ones – it is this 'iatrogenesis' that both manifests and impacts profoundly.

The book contributes to the understanding of peer support interventions in custody, specifically peer-led induction and how such a power-sharing initiatives can interact with the experience of imprisonment and the pains of imprisonment at the key times of transfer, transition and adaptation to both a new and open prison. Unlike previous studies on penal power and responsibilisation, this book applies the concept of institutional iatrogenesis to demonstrate how interventions intended to support prisoners may actively contribute to their distress. It is clear that prison is a painful experience, both historically and in the present day, and throughout, the book explored how the process was experienced by those who were imprisoned first and foremost. In doing so, it considered the challenges, thoughts and feelings they experienced in the early day of custody post-transfer and how peer-led induction interacted with that. It demonstrated the considerable strain on mental health experienced by those entering a new custodial establishment, which is a clear indicator of transition as a stressful experience. In doing so, it further considered the pains associated with imprisonment and these processes, building upon earlier theorisation of Sykes (1958) and Crewe (2011a, 2011b), in the context of forgotten pains. These are conceptualised as the pain of transfer and adaptation/adjustment, which are founded on conditions of *entry shock* and a *fear of the unknown*. In doing so, it elicited perceptions of those staff involved in the implementation and delivery of the intervention, revealing a number of key themes and considerations that interact with the efficacy of the intervention. It also considered the organisational challenges that threaten the efficacy of the intervention, considering what support prisoners should be offered during entry and adaptation to the prison and contrasting against the reality of what is experienced. The reality was often captured through the emergent themes of self-interest and disinterest among mentors and staff. These all-underpinned issues relate to negative mental health and well-being outcomes among prisoners. The book has been able to identify and explore a range of structural impediments to peer-led induction. These related to the complex construct of institutional managerialism, with the entanglement of ineffective management and resistant staff cultures interacting to divert focus away from helping those who are imprisoned to better adapt and alleviate mental health and well-being issues in the early days in the new establishment.

Power is a concept that is deeply embedded throughout. Emerging from the empirical study is the notion that reconfigured penal power through the power-sharing between prisoners and staff in peer-led induction challenges occupational discourses around the identity of the prison officer and how the prison officers should 'carry out their duties'. These issues are indicative of a 'tick-box culture' that prevents prison officers from connecting with offenders and underpins peers and staff fulfiling management and self-serving objectives and goals. Furthermore, the application of power through strategies of responsibilisation reveals the model as failing to employ a needs-driven approach to induction. Responsibilisation is operationalised as a 'smoke-screen' at times, due to a lack of staff and mentor visibility in the induction process and lack of engagement with inductees. This power-infused responsibilisation interacts closely with the concept of 'tightness'. It underpins the feelings of anxiety and stress of induction mentees and undermines the potential for the intervention to have meaningful engagement, alleviating the mental distress of new prisoners. How power, in the form of this power-sharing initiative, manifests in the experience of transfer and adaptation is further demonstrated through the range of conceptualisations, concerning self-serving motivations, paradoxical social support and the abuse and misuse of power. All this culminates in ramping up the thermostat of penal tightness for those subject to the peer-led induction. It conceptualises peer-led induction as a form of 'intervention-itis', signifying the saturation of such schemes in the prison estate as a quick fix or quick win for the institution to paper over the cracks that exist. As such, there is limited thought in the design and implementation phase, which serves to have deleterious impacts upon prisoner mental health and well-being, thus increasing the tightness of the penal experience.

When considering these in their totality, peer-led induction is positioned as an intervention plagued by a lack of a sound theoretical and evaluative footing, one which would provide the aim of the programme in the form of an efficient Programme Theory, especially in terms of evaluation and the application of evaluation. As such, it has been important to establish the role of Programme Theory and its importance in the design, implementation and delivery of peer support interventions broadly, and more specifically peer-led induction, especially in an age where penal policy has seen a plethora of interventions and schemes thrown at addressing fundamental issues stemming from the conditions of imprisonment in England and Wales, with the clamour to do so precluding the devil in the detail.

This final chapter is both reflective and forward thinking in nature with the empirical grounding throughout the book and these ideas, arguably transferable organisationally beyond just a peer led induction, to other peer interventions and other prisons and security categories. It firstly reflects on the key challenges that peer-led induction faces while considering how these can be addressed. In doing so, it draws upon the conceptualisations advanced, before considering how it can be situated within a framework of policy and intervention change and challenges the makers of penal policy to double down on the mantra that 'prisoners lives matter'. It encourages them to be bold in doing so, by accepting the flaws and issues identified, but doing so both critically and constructively to bring about change that produces the best possible outcomes for the mental health and well-being of the many men transferring and transitioning to the final phase of their custodial journey and life outside of the prison walls.

Where Do We Go From Here? Key Intervention Challenges and Changes

What is clear is that there are a number of pertinent iatrogenic outcomes that compromise the design, implementation and delivery of an effective and needs-driven peer-led induction. The chapter now turns to identifying these key challenges and considers ways to address them.

Managerialism and Staff Culture

A key is the notion that 'good programme management is the key to successful implementation of [offending behaviour] programmes' (Hollin & Palmer, 2006, p. 10). This is also true in relation to peer-led induction. There was the presence of a resistant culture to management, born out of issues relating to trust and how management were perceived as more orientated towards fulfiling their management targets and delivering a top-down approach. This was conceptualised as being indicative of a tick-box culture, dominating and pervading what should be an intervention to deliver positive outcomes in relation to the mental health and well-being of the mentee rather than managerialist priorities and targets. This approach created a wariness of management from staff who felt disenfranchised as a result of this approach and as such were much more resistant to sharing and converting knowledge that could have been used in a bottom-up approach to the benefit of the peer-led induction, thus improving outcomes for both prisoner mentees and management, who struggled to engage their staff to convert. There needs to be much more synergy between management. Clear lines of communication between both parties – with a greater level of support for and recognition of the knowledge and experience of those staff on the ground and the challenges they face, resource support and the incentivisation of the intervention – would garner buy in among the staff and increasing the legitimacy of the management. Advances in this area, as discussed earlier, would underpin a workforce that is much more conducive with both converting and sharing knowledge with management to make for a more effective provision.

Selection and Training (Staff and Peer Security)

Of prominence was the motivations of peer support workers and staff in relation to the peer-led induction. There was the notion expressed by the ex-prisoner sample that the peer support workers engaged in activities that were in breach of prison security measures and that they were in the positions they were to facilitate these outcomes or to benefit in some way by accessing material goods or those staff members involved in the ROTL process. This highlighted the motivations as self-serving and as not embracing what should be an altruistic endeavour to provide support to those in need. Similarly, staff reported issues about staff members resistant to the ethos of power-sharing in the peer-led induction and how staff involved in the inductions enacted the role of a prison officer. To these staff members, it challenged an occupational culture where there is a historic understanding of how the prison officer should 'do prison' and symbolised that shift to softer power. Staff members undermined the effectiveness of the provision when having to work in induction by conforming to their own person ethos and ignoring the culture of power-sharing. All these issues point towards problems surrounding effective selection and training of peer support workers and staff who come into contact with the provision of induction. While necessary pools of those prisoners and staff with the requisite experience, ability and skill may be in short supply in the prison setting, there, nonetheless, needs to be some effort to adopt a criteria and resources to embrace and develop the core values of a power-sharing endeavour of peer-led induction.

Empowerment and Support

As documented, responsibilisation is a key strategy of the open prison. However, responsibilising strategies are a source of anxiety, stress and the pains of transfer and adaptation at a time when they are experienced very acutely. Prisoners found themselves almost cut adrift by the notion of having to find their own way while also contending with what this book recognises as the process of double liminality. Often, this lack of engagement was perceived as a lack of visibility and interest by staff and peers and was conceptualised as an abuse or misuse of power. These responsibilising measures exist with coercion in the form of regression to closed conditions or lack of progress within the open prison, with this fear causing immense distress among prisoners, captured as 'tightness' in their experience of imprisonment. Responsibilisation is intended to enable and empower, but, in reality, it has crippling effects that are supported by perceived apathy among staff and peer support workers. The combination of these elements is shown as leading to a paradoxical outcome, whereby prisons sought out the support and advice they needed to navigate this time of transition from networks of fellow prisoners, rather than peer support workers and induction staff, which undermines the existence of the intervention itself. The responsibilising strategies of open prison would arguably be better suited to being operationalised once a supportive, responsive, needs-based and relational induction is completed, one that revolves around altruism, effective communication and dissemination of information and once the prisoner suitably adapted. Responsibilisation is not a word to be banded around to mask or excuse deficiencies in these areas.

Design, Implementation, Delivery: Monitoring and Evaluation

'Intervention-itis' plays a role in the compromise of the intervention. The clamour to get interventions out there has led to arguably less robust, less evidence- and theory-based interventions to be put in place to plug the gaps in a prison system fit to burst under the strain of its issues. The response is a plethora of such interventions, symbolic of 'intervention-itis'. Something is not better than nothing if that something does not achieve its intended aims and consequently produces iatrogenic outcomes. This is what peer-led induction does; it produces iatrogenic harm. There is a lack of sufficient focus on Programme Theory in peer-led induction to develop it to a level where it both meets its intended aims and objectives and is free from the shackles of iatrogenic outcomes that diminish it. For all the rhetoric and literature that exists about the rigours of accredited programmes, the fact remains that peer-led induction is not one, alongside other interventions within the walls of prisons that those who are imprisoned engage with. There remains a huge void between Offending Behaviour (OB) interventions and others that are not offending behaviour orientated, as well as non-accredited, with the latter appearing to be cut adrift. They are devoid of the same rigour in relation to promoting best and effective practice and from receiving the diligence that accreditation brings, as introduced earlier, especially surrounding evaluation. Delivering and maintaining effective practice across all interventions, including peer-led induction, must be a focus if the principles of effective practice are to be translated into action. Programme accreditation and audit are key to ensuring that interventions embody the principles of effective practice introduced earlier and are effective through quality delivery. Yet these are not applied here as it is neither an offending behaviour programme nor accredited. Ultimately, by neglecting these areas in the realm of non-offending behaviour interventions, those who are imprisoned are also being neglected. This neglects prisoner outcomes surrounding health and well-being in favour of a disproportionate focus on outcomes surrounding re-offending rates. Arguably, the inference is that delivering the best possible interventions for those who are imprisoned with the highest possible standards is not a consideration when it does not concern the field of recidivism; otherwise, this book and many other critiques of penal interventions would not be written, at least not with the level of issues they elucidate. By not focusing on Programme Theory or accrediting in regard to peer-led induction, there are not the conditions for giving the maximum focus available to the peer-led induction. Theory and accreditation are not enough alone. The issues identified are not individual cogs; they need to be addressed as part of a bigger structure. There remains the potential for Programme Theory and accreditation to become a tick-box exercise too rather than the next golden goose to improve everything.

Where Do We Go From Here? Future Research

It has been established that the transition and adaptation to the way of life within the open prison estate comes with a range of challenges that impact the mental health and well-being of those that encounter them. Peer-led induction is a support to try and mitigate these by helping prisoners navigate an environment that is complex but not unequivocally successful. The already complex nature of open prisons has changed during the time between the empirical research, with there for example, being newer policies regarding aspects of the regime. Previously, prisoners had to complete a 'lay down period', months of monitoring and assessment before being allowed to progress through various stages of community release. There were other restrictive rules too regarding work placements. However, these changed in late 2019, including eligibility for Resettlement Day Release (RDR) starting from the point of transfer; there is no longer a restriction on ROTL for the first 3 months following transfer to open conditions and prisoners are now eligible for ROTL once all sentence planning and risk management procedures have taken place (Prison Reform Trust, 2019b). COVID-19 hit also open prisons hard as they were unable to carry out their main purpose of preparing prisoners for release through large numbers of the population of these prions working and developing skills off-site in the community, and there is a legacy of the institutional changes to the present day, which impact the experience of imprisonment. All these factors represent more layers to the experience of imprisonment and more opportunity for psychological distress for the prisoner. As such, the further study of the open prison today and reflecting these conditions and their legacy in structural and institutional change in the experience of those imprisoned who have experienced them would be welcomed to fully encapsulate and reconcile conditions and experience of them. A larger sample across multiple open prison sites across the open prison estate in England and Wales would also assist with extending the comprehensiveness and representativeness of study into this field. Furthermore, by conducting this research in the prison estate, as a full ethnographic endeavour, there will be the opportunity to engage with prisoners being received into the establishment at the pinch points of transfer and transition. Doing so, alongside a longitudinal approach, when carrying out further study in this construct would allow for the charting the prisoners at the time of reception and pre-induction and then again after the induction process, allowing for a greater depth to study in this realm. Finally, self-serving motivations have been a perception levied at both peer support workers and staff involved in the induction. However, it could also signify that the same self-serving motivations exist within the peer mentees as to why they wish to paint the peer support workers and staff in this manner. One voice that is not represented in the study is the voice of the peer support workers. Moving forward, study in this realm should seek where possible to ensure that all actors involved in the process of induction are given a voice. Their perceptions of the staff they share power with and those mentees that they interact with are valuable to supporting a more rounded perspective. The same can be said for the prison management, who are similarly perceived in a negative manner by the staff sample. This would allow for a much more in-depth consideration of staff and management cultures, motivations and dynamics.

Where Do We Go From Here? Situating for Future Policy and Intervention Change

The Areas of Research Interest (ARI) document (Ministry of Justice, 2020) is part of the Ministry of Justice's (MOJ) ambition to put evidence at the heart of the justice system. It is an illustrative guiding document focusing on the key strategic areas in which the MOJ has indicated the need for an increase in the available evidence base. I utilise this document as a framework within which to situate the book and its study and demonstrate its applicability organisationally so that it abundantly clear to those in policy of its relationship. This ARI summarises the MOJ's evidence needs, aligned with the department's strategic objectives for the system. These objectives directly relating to the prison system include:

- Ensuring that prisons are decent, safe and productive places to live and work.
- Protecting the public from harm.
- Reducing rates of reoffending and improve life chances.

(MOJ, 2020)

While there is already an evidence base for these specified areas, the MOJ recognises that the penal landscape is ever changing and the need to continually develop the evidence base is ongoing. There are a plethora of areas requiring this attention to expand the evidence base, yet focus is applied here to identifying those that this book informs.

It is expressed that the MOJ seek to ensure that prisons are decent, safe and productive places to live and work as a core aim. Key aims that this study feeds into include MOJ aims to:

- Provide decent, safe and secure accommodation that supports individuals.
- Reduce levels of violence and self-harm and develop the evidence on what structures and interventions can help improve outcomes for individuals in prison. In doing so, it requires them to better understand pathways, what works for whom and when, to ensure that interventions and support are targeted and timely.

(MOJ, 2020)

As such, they employ research questions, reflective of their evidence priorities which also relate to the purpose and intended outcomes of this body of work, including:

- How effective are different prison types, categories and functions such as reception in meeting their core objectives?
- What works across our prisons to increase safety and security and reduce levels of violence?
- How can we effectively balance prison and secure establishment approaches to safety and security, with the delivery of other services and initiatives in prisons?

(MOJ, 2020)

More specifically, it looks at services and interventions posing the questions below to which this book adds insight:

- How can services and therapeutic interventions, such as training, peer and family relationship, support and improve outcomes?
- How can we better understand the impact of interventions delivered in prisons?
- What works, for whom, to support effective transition and resettlement?

(MOJ, 2020)

In the health and well-being sphere, it directly addresses and resonates most with the investigation of:

- What works to reduce levels of self-harm and self-inflicted death in prisons for different individuals and groups?
- How can mentoring, peer support and staff relationships help in reducing self-harm?

(MOJ, 2020)

As such, it is possible to relate and situate the research drawn upon and the narrative presented within these organisational and institutional aims and objectives. Policymakers need to embrace the notion that no single regime, or type of regime, is perfect for all prisoners or even for the same prisoner at various points in their life, and this needs to be factored in better to deliver a needs-driven model. There's no silver bullet to the complex set of issues facing people transferring to open prison. Different things will work in different circumstances. This in itself illustrates the need for embracing newer approaches. According to Curtis and Edwards (2019, p. 358), a more progressive strategy is needed, as 'most successful initiatives have been driven from the frontline in active collaboration with the individuals involved' and 'placing the user at the centre of service design will not only dictate the information required and who needs access to it [. . .] but will improve transparency and accountability'. A peer-led induction model that adopts these concepts and employs evidence such as this book's contents would arguably go a long way towards informing addressing the majority of the concerns raised during the study. How this can be achieved in policy is not the purpose of this book. Rather, it is the intent to provide insight into the experience of the intervention and how it is operationalised and implemented to provide and support and evidence base for change.

This book and its contents are an invitation to policymakers within the criminal justice system to be bold when considering what works and what doesn't: to be brave and gravitate away from cherry-picking whereby they pick only the best people or things from a group so that only people or things that are less good remain. In a book that has at length discussed self-serving motivations and enduring issues in the penal system, these issues are evident in the policymakers too. Despite seeking to gather evidence to form a basis upon which to act, the penal system is still in crisis. Seemingly, there are issues with the evidence base being collated or, rather, how it is used and translated into practise to address the issues prisons and prisoners face every day. As such, this is a crucial juncture for this book to provide a richer understanding of peer-led induction and its interaction with the experience of imprisonment at the crucial time of transfer, transition and adaptation to the open prison estate. The analysis in this book challenges the assumption that all interventions in prison settings inherently provide support. By demonstrating how peer-led induction can unintentionally reinforce distress, power imbalances and psychological strain, this book presents a case for rethinking the design and evaluation of prison interventions.

If interventions lack clear theoretical grounding, structured oversight and robust evaluation mechanisms, they risk becoming counterproductive. If prison interventions are to be meaningful, they must move beyond the rhetoric of support and instead be rooted in evidence, reflexivity and genuine engagement with the needs of those they claim to serve. Anything less risks perpetuating the very harms they seek to alleviate.

References

Abu-Jarad, I., Yusof, N., & Nikbin, D. (2010). A review paper on organizational culture and organizational performance. *International Journal of Business and Social Science*, *1*, 26–46.

Adair, D. (2005). *Peer support programs within prisons*. Dissertation. University of Tasmania School of Sociology and Social Work.

Adams, K. (1992). Adjusting to prison life. *Crime and Justice*, *16*, 275–359.

Adams, R., Bessant, J., & Phelps, R. (2006). Innovation management measurement: A review. *International Journal of Management Reviews*, *8*(1), 21–47.

Adatia, R. (2010). Offender mental health. https://www.jsna.info/sites/jsna.info/files/JSNA%20Westminster%202010%20Offender%20Mental%20Health.pdf

Addis, M. E. (2011). *Invisible men: Men's inner lives and the consequences of silence*. Macmillan.

Adler, P. A., & Adler, P. (2011). *The tender cut: Inside the hidden world of self-injury*. NYU Press.

Al-Adaileh, R. M., & Al-Atawi, M. S. (2011). Organizational culture impact on knowledge exchange: Saudi Telecom context. *Journal of Knowledge Management*, *15*(2), 212–230.

Alder, S. (n.d.). Quote. https://www.goodreads.com/quotes/683558-most-misunderstandings-in-the-world-could-be-avoided-if-people

Alford, C. F. (2000). What would it matter if everything Foucault said about prison were wrong: 'Discipline and Punish' after twenty years. *Theory and Society*, *29*(1), 125–146.

Alhady, S., Sawal, M., Idris, A., Azmi, A., & Zakaria, Z. (2011). Knowledge sharing behavior and individual factors: A relationship study in the I-class environment. In *International proceedings of economics development and research*. IACSIT Press.

Allison, E. (2017, December 20). There's a mental health crisis in our prisons, yet the justice secretary is silent. *The Guardian*. https://www.theguardian.com/commentisfree/2017/dec/20/prisoners-mental-healthself-harm-deaths-jails-liverpool

Annison, H., & Condry, R. (2018). *The pains of indeterminate imprisonment for family members findings and recommendations: Extended report*. University of Southampton.

Antojado, D., & McPhee, T. (2024). Move over and make space for lived experience criminology: Why we do "lived experience". *Journal of Criminology*. https://doi.org/10.1177/26338076241286534

Aresti, A., Darke, S., & Manlow, D. (2016). Bridging the gap: Giving public voice to prisoners and former prisoners through research activism. *Prison Service Journal*, *224*, 3–13.

Arnold, H., Liebling, A., & Tait, S. (2007). Prison officers and prison culture. In Y. Jewkes (Ed.), *Handbook on prisons* (pp. 501–525). Willan Publishing.

Arseneault, C., Plourde, C., & Alain, M. (2016). Evaluating a prison-based intervention program: Approaches and challenges. *Canadian Journal of Program Evaluation*, *31*(1), 61–81.

Asrar-ul-Haq, M., & Anwar, S. (2016). A systematic review of knowledge management and knowledge sharing: Trends, issues, and challenges. *Cogent Business & Management*, *3*(1).

Ballesteros-Pena, A. (2018). Responsibilisation and female imprisonment in contemporary penal policy: 'Respect Modules' ('Módulos de Respeto') in Spain. *Punishment & Society*, *20*(4), 458–476.

Bandura, A. (1986). *Social foundations of thought and action: A social cognitive theory*. Prentice Hall.

Baxter Magolda, M. B. (2004). Evolution of a constructivist conceptualization of epistemological reflection. *Educational Psychologist*, *39*(1), 31–42.

Baybutt, M., Dooris, M., & Farrier, A. (2019). Growing health in UK prison settings. *Health Promotion International*, *34*(4), 792–802.

Bean, P. (1981). *Punishment: A philosophical and criminological inquiry*. Robertson.

Bennett, J. (2016). *The working lives of prison managers: Global change, local culture and individual agency in the late modern prison*. Palgrave Macmillan.

Berger, P. L., & Luckman, T. (1967). *The social construction of reality: A treatise on the sociology of knowledge*. Anchor.

Beyens, K., Kennes, P., Snacken, S., & Tournal, H. (2015). The craft of doing qualitative research in prisons. *Crime and Justice Journal*, *4*(1), 66–78.

Bhatti, W., Waris, S., Zaheer, A., & Rehman, K. (2011). The effect of commitment and motivation on human talent and its contribution to organizational performance. *Management & Marketing Challenges for the Knowledge Society*, *6*, 471–482.

Blaauw, E., Schilder, F., & van de Lande, S. (1998). Prevention of suicides in the Dutch CJS. In A. Liebling (Ed.), *Deaths of offenders: The hidden side of justice* (pp. 201–223). Waterside Press.

Blagden, N., & Perrin, C. (2014). *An overview of peer support in prison: An internal report for NOMS*. https://www.researchgate.net/publication/322699359_An_overview_of_peer_support_in_prison_An_internal_report_for_NOMS

Boothby, M. (2011). Insiders' views of their role: Toward their training. *Canadian Journal of Criminology and Criminal Justice*, *53*(4), 424–448.

Borkman, T. J. (1990). Experiential, professional, and lay frames of reference. In T. J. Powell (Ed.), *Working with self-help* (pp. 3–30). National Association of Social Work.

Bosworth, M. (2007). Creating the responsible prisoner: Federal admission and orientation packs. *Punishment & Society*, *9*(1), 67–85.

Bowling, B. (2011). Transnational criminology and the globalization of harm production. In M. Bosworth & C. Hoyle (Eds.), *What is criminology?* (pp. 361–379). Oxford University Press.

Bowring, J. (Ed.). (1843). *The works of Jeremy Bentham*. William Tait. https://oll.libertyfund.org/title/bentham-works-of-jeremy-bentham-11-vols

Boyce, I., Hunter, G., & Hough, M. (2009). *St Giles trust peer advice project: An evaluation*. St Giles Trust.

Boyle, D. (2021). *Tickbox*. Little, Brown Books Group.

Bradley, K. (2009). *The Bradley Report: Lord Bradley's review of people with mental health problems or learning disabilities in the criminal justice system.* https://lx.iriss.org.uk/sites/default/files/resources/The%20Bradley%20report.pdf

Brown, G., & Bos, E. (2017). 'We were there too': There is much to learn from embedding auto/biography in the knowing and doing of prison research. *Methodological Innovations, 10*(2). https://doi.org/10.1177/2059799117724039

Bucher, S. V., Chreim, S., Langley, A., & Reay, T. (2016). Contestation about collaboration: Discursive boundary work among professions. *Organization Studies, 37*(4), 497–522.

Buck, G. (2018). The core conditions of peer mentoring. *Criminology and Criminal Justice, 18*(2), 190–206.

Buck, G. (2020). *Peer mentoring in criminal justice*. Routledge.

Buck, G., Tomczak, P., Harriott, P., Page, R., Bradley, K., Nash, M., & Wainwright, L. (2023). Prisoners on prisons: Experiences of peer-delivered suicide prevention work. *Incarceration, 4*. https://doi.org/10.1177/26326663231172023

Bulman, M. (2019, July 25). Mental health support failings fuel rise in self-harm and suicide in custody, say experts. *The Independent*. https://www.independent.co.uk/news/uk/home-news/mental-health-prison-selfharm-suicide-offenders-a9020396.html

Caddle, D. (1995). *A survey of the prisoner escort and custody service provided by Group 4 and by SCS*. Home Office.

Cahill, T. J., Jessell, J. C., & Horne, A. M. (1979). Peer and professional counsellors: Prisoners' preferences and evaluations. *Criminal Justice and Behavior, 6*, 400–415.

Caird, R. (1974). *A good and useful life: Imprisonment in Britain today*. HartDavis, MacGibbon.

Carlen, P. (1994). Why study women's imprisonment? Or anyone else's?: An indefinite article. In D. King & M. Maguire (Eds.), *Prisons in context* (pp. 131–140). Clarendon Press.

Carlile, P. R. (2002). A pragmatic view of knowledge and boundaries: Boundary objects in new product development. *Organization Science, 13*(4), 442–455.

Carlile, P. R. (2004). Transferring, translating, and transforming: An integrative framework for managing knowledge across boundaries. *Organization Science, 15*(5), 555–568.

Cavaliere, V., Lombardi, S., & Giustiniano, L. (2015). Knowledge sharing in knowledge intensive manufacturing firms. An empirical study of its enablers. *Journal of Knowledge Management, 19*(6), 1124–1145.

Cheliotis, L. K. (2008). Reconsidering the effectiveness of temporary release: A systematic review. *Aggression and Violent Behavior, 13*(3), 153–168.

Chiseri-Strater, E. (1996). Turning in upon ourselves: Positionality, subjectivity, and reflexivity in case study and ethnographic research. In P. Mortensen & G. E. Kirsch (Eds.), *Ethics and responsibility in qualitative studies of literacy* (pp. 115–133). NCTE.

Clemmer, D. (1940). *The prison community*. Christopher.

Cohen, S. (1988). Western crime models in the third world: Benign or malignant. In *Against criminology new Brunswick New Jersey: Transaction*. Original paper presented University of Ibadan, Nigeria, 1980.

Cohen, S. (1998). *Against criminology*. Routledge.

Cohen, S. (2001). *States of denial: A new perspective*. Blackwell.

Cohen, L., Manion, L., & Morrison, K. (2011). *Research methods in education*. Routledge.

Cohen, A. P., & Rapport, N. (1995). *Questions of consciousness* (pp. 1–18). Routledge.

Cohen, S., & Taylor, L. (1981). *Psychological survival: The experience of long-term imprisonment*. Penguin.

Cohen, S., & Wills, T. A. (1985). Stress, social support, and the buffering hypothesis. *Psychological Bulletin*, *98*(2), 310.

Contu, A., & Willmott, H. (2003). Re-embedding situatedness: The importance of power relations in learning theory. *Organization Science*, *14*(3), 283–296.

Cook, J., McClure, S., Koutsenok, I., & Lord, S. (2008). The implementation of inmate mentor programs in the correctional treatment system as an innovative approach. *Journal of Teaching in the Addictions*, *7*(2), 123–132.

Cook-Sather, A. (2006). Newly betwixt and between: Revising liminality in the context of a teacher preparation program. *Anthropology & Education Quarterly*, *37*(2), 110–127.

Cox, C., & Marland, H. (2018). Broken minds and beaten bodies: Cultures of harm and the management of mental illness in mid- to late nineteenth-century English and Irish prisons. *Social History of Medicine: The Journal of the Society for the Social History of Medicine*, *31*(4), 688–710.

Coyle, A. (1994). *The prisons we deserve*. HarperCollins.

Crapanzano, V. (1977). On the writing of ethnography. *Dialectical Anthropology*, *2*, 69–73.

Crawley, E. (2004). *Doing prison work: The public and private lives of prison officers*. Willan Publishing.

Crawley, E. (2005). Institutional thoughtlessness in prisons and its impacts on the day-to-day prison lives of elderly men. *Journal of Contemporary Criminal Justice*, *21*(4), 350–363.

Crawley, E., & Crawley, P. (2007). Understanding prison officers: Culture, cohesion and conflict. In J. Bennett, B. Crewe, & A. Wahidin (Eds.), *Understanding prison staff* (pp. 134–152). Routledge.

Cressey, D. R. (1960). The theory of differential association: An introduction. *Social Problems*, *8*, 2.

Crewe, B. (2007). Power, adaptation and resistance in a late-modern men's prison. *British Journal of Criminology*, *47*(2), 256–275.

Crewe, B. (2009). *The prisoner society: Power, adaptation and social life in an English prison*. Oxford University Press.

Crewe, B. (2011a). Depth, weight, tightness: Revisiting the pains of imprisonment. *Punishment & Society*, *13*(5), 509–529.

Crewe, B. (2011b). Soft power in prison: Implications for staff–prisoner relationships, liberty and legitimacy. *European Journal of Criminology*, *8*(6), 455–468.

Crewe, B. (2015). Inside the belly of the beast: Understanding the experience of imprisonment. *The International Journal for Crime, Justice and Social Democracy*, *4*(1), 50–65.

Crewe, B., & Ievins, A. (2020). 'Tightness', recognition and penal power. *Punishment & Society*, *23*(1). https://doi.org/10.1177/1462474520928115

Crewe, B., & Liebling, A. (2017). Reconfiguring penal power. In A. Liebling, S. Maruna, & L. McAra (Eds.), *The Oxford handbook of criminology* (6th ed.). Oxford University Press.

Crewe, B., Liebling, A., & Hulley, S. (2014). Heavy–light, absent–present: Rethinking the 'weight' of imprisonment. *British Journal of Sociology*, *65*(3), 387–410.

Criminal Justice Alliance (CJA). (2019). *Changes from within: Insights from people with lived experience working to improve the criminal justice system*. http://www.criminaljusticealliance.org

Cullen, F. T. (1994). Social support as an organizing concept for criminology: Presidential address to the academy of criminal justice sciences. *Justice Quarterly*, *11*(4), 527–559.

Curtis, S., & Edwards, J. (2019). Improving public services by sharing the right information. *Public Money & Management*, *39*(5), 355–358.

Czarnecka, B., & Massaro, M. R. (2021). Why do students dislike research methods modules and what to do about it? In *Teaching marketing* (pp. 201–222). Edward Elgar Publishing.

Danks, K., & Bradley, A. (2018). Negotiating barriers: Prisoner and staff perspectives on mental wellbeing in the open prison setting. *Journal of Criminal Psychology*, *8*(1), 3–19.

Darley, D., Davies, B., Earle, R., Honeywell, D., & Schreeche-Powell, E. (2023). Creating convict criminology in the UK: a response to Aresti, Darke and Ross from members of the British Convict Criminology Group. *Justice, Power and Resistance*, *6*(3), 328–338.

Davenport, T., De Long, D., & Beers, M. (1998). Successful knowledge management projects. *Sloan Management Review*, *39*(2), 43–57.

Davidoff, F., Dixon-Woods, M., Leviton, L., & Michie, S. (2015). Demystifying theory and its use in improvement. *BMJ Quality and Safety*, *24*(3), 228–238.

Davidson, L., Bellamy, C., Guy, K., & Miller, R. (2012). Peer support among persons with severe mental illnesses: A review of evidence and experience. *World Psychiatry: Official Journal of the World Psychiatric Association (WPA)*, *11*(2), 123–128.

Davies, R. (1966). *Dedicated follower of fashion*. Sittin' on My Sofa [Vinyl]. Pye Records.

Davies, B. (1994). The Swansea listener scheme: Views from the prison landings. *The Howard Journal of Criminal Justice*, *33*(2), 125–135.

Davies, W. (2015). Unique position: Dual identities as prison researcher and ex-prisoner. In *The Palgrave handbook of prison ethnography* (pp. 463–478). Palgrave Macmillan UK.

Davies, B., & Harré, R. (1990). Positioning: The discursive production of selves. *Journal for the Theory of Social Behaviour*, *20*(1), 43–63.

De Laine, M. (2000). *Fieldwork, participation and practice: Ethics and dilemmas in qualitative research*. Sage.

De Vigianni, N. (2006). Surviving prison: Exploring prisons social life as a determinant of health. *International Journal of Prisoner Health*, *2*(2), 71–89.

Dean, M. (1999). *Governmentality: Power and rule in modern society*. Sage.

Delveaux, K., & Blanchette, K. (2000). *Results of an evaluation of the peer support program at Nova Institution for women*. Correctional Service Canada.

Dembele, L., Nathan, S., Carter, A., Costello, J., Hodgins, M., Singh, R., Martin, B., & Cullen, P. (2024). Researching with lived experience: A shared critical reflection between co-researchers. *International Journal of Qualitative Methods*, *23*. https://doi.org/10.1177/16094069241257945

Deshpandé, R., Farley, J. U., & Webster, F. E., Jr. (1993). Corporate culture, customer orientation, and innovativeness in Japanese firms: A quadrad analysis. *Journal of Marketing*, *57*(1), 23–37.

Devilly, G., Sorbello, L., Eccleston, L., & Ward, T. (2005). Prison-based peer education schemes. *Aggression and Violent Behavior*, *10*, 219–240.

Dickens, C. (1842/1883). *American notes*. John W. Lowell Company.

Dickson-Swift, V., James, E. L., Kippen, S., & Liamputtong, P. (2007). Doing sensitive research: What challenges do qualitative researchers face? *Qualitative Research*, *7*(3), 327–353.

Dilulio, J. J., Jr. (1987). *Governing prisons: A comparative study of correctional management*. Free Press.

Drake, D. H., Earle, R., & Sloan, J. (Eds.). (2015). *The Palgrave handbook of prison ethnography* (pp. 252–270). Palgrave Macmillan.

Durcan, G. (2008). *From the inside*. Experiences of Prison Mental Health Care, Sainsbury Centre for Mental Health.

Durcan, G., Saunders, S., Gadsby, B., & Hazard, A. (2014). *The Bradley Report five years on: An independent review of progress to date and priorities for further development*. Centre for Mental Health.

Dwyer, S. C., & Buckle, J. L. (2009). The space between: On being an insider-outsider in qualitative research. *International Journal of Qualitative Methods*, *8*(1), 54–63.

Dysvik, A., Buch, R., & Kuvaas, B. (2013). Knowledge donating and knowledge collecting: The moderating roles of social and economic LMX. *The Leadership & Organization Development Journal*, *36*, 35–53.

Earle, R. (2014). Insider and out. *Qualitative Inquiry*, *20*(4), 429–438.

Earle, E. (2016). What is convict criminology. *Rod Earle*. https://www.open.ac.uk/researchcentres/herc/blog/what-convict-criminology

Earle, R. (2018). Convict criminology in England: Developments and dilemmas. *British Journal of Criminology*, *58*(6), 1499–1516. https://doi.org/10.1093/bjc/azy016

Earle, R., Darley, D., Davies, B., Honeywell, D., & Schreeche-Powell, E. (2023). Convict criminology without guarantees: Proposing hard labour for an unfinished criminology. In A. Liebling, S. Maruna, & L. McAra (Eds.), *The Oxford handbook of criminology* (7th ed., pp. 911–932). Oxford University Press.

Ehly, S. W., & Vazquez, E. G. (1998). Peer counselling. In K. Topping & S. W. Ehly (Eds.), *Peer assisted learning*. Routledge.

Eide, P., & Allen, C. B. (2005). Recruiting transcultural qualitative research participants: A conceptual model. *International Journal of Qualitative Methods*, *4*(2), 44–56.

Elias, N. (1978). *The civilizing process*. Urizen Books.

Elias, N. (1984). Knowledge and power: An interview by Peter Ludes. In N. Stehr & M. Volker (Eds.), *Society and knowledge: Contemporary perspectives in the sociology of knowledge* (pp. 251–291). : Transaction Publishers.

Ely, M., Anzul, M., Friedman, T., Garner, D., & Steinmetz, A. (1991). *Doing qualitative research: Circles within circles*. Falmer Press.

England, K. V. L. (1994). Getting personal: Reflexivity, positionality, and feminist research. *The Professional Geographer*, *46*(1), 80–89.

Engstrand, Å.-K., & Enberg, C. (2020). The power in positionings: A Foucauldian approach to knowledge integration processes. *Management Learning*, *51*(3), 336–352. https://doi.org/10.1177/1350507620904307

Enosh, G., & Ben-Ari, A. (2016, March). Reflexivity: The creation of liminal spaces – Researchers, participants, and research encounters. *Qualitative Health Research*, *26*(4), 578–584. https://doi.org/10.1177/1049732315587878

Ericson, R. V., & Haggerty, K. D. (1997). *Policing the risk society*. Clarendon Press.

Esmée Fairbairn Foundation. (2004). Rethinking crime and punishment. https://esmeefairbairn.org.uk/our-aims/learning-and-insights/rethinking-crime-punishment/

Etherington, K. (1996). The counsellor as researcher: Boundary issues and critical dilemmas. *British Journal of Guidance and Counselling*, *24*, 339–346.

Exworthy, T., Samele, C., Urquia, N., & Forrester, A. (2012). Asserting prisoners' right to health: Progressing beyond equivalence. *Psychiatric Services*, *63*(3), 270–275.

Faraj, S., & Yan, A. (2009). Boundary work in knowledge teams. *Journal of Applied Psychology*, *94*(3), 604–617.

Fazel, S., & Danesh, J. (2002). Serious mental disorder in 23,000 prisoners: A systematic review of 62 surveys. *Lancet*, *359*(9306), 545–550.

Fazel, S., Grann, M., Kling, B., & Hawton, K. (2011). Prison suicide in 12 countries: An ecological study of 861 suicides during 2003–2007. *Social Psychiatry and Psychiatric Epidemiology*, *46*, 191–195.

Fenge, L. A., Oakley, L., Taylor, B., & Beer, S. (2019). The impact of sensitive research on the researcher: Preparedness and positionality. *International Journal of Qualitative Methods*, *18*. https://doi.org/10.1177/1609406919893161

Feynman, R. (1974). Cargo cult science. *Engineering and Science*, *37*(7), 10–13.

Fletcher, D., & Batty, E. (2012). *Offender Peer Intervention: What do we know?* Centre for Regional Economic and Social Research. https://www4.shu.ac.uk/research/cresr/sites/shu.ac.uk/files/offenderpeerinterventions.pdf

Fong, C., Ooi, K., Tan, B., Lee, V., & Chong, A. Y. (2011). HRM practices and knowledge sharing: An empirical study. *International Journal of Manpower*, *32*, 704–723.

Forsey, M. (2010). Ethnography as participant listening. *Ethnography*, *11*(4), 558–572.

Foucault, M. (1975). *Surveiller et punir: Naissance de la prison*. Gallimard.

Foucault, M. (1977). *Discipline and punish: The birth of the prison*. Allen Lane.

Foucault, M. (1988). Technologies of the self. In L. H. Martin, H. Gutman, & P. H. Hutton (Eds.), *Technologies of the self: A seminar with Michel Foucault* (pp. 16–49). University of Massachusetts Press.

Franke, H. (1995). *The emancipation of prisoners: A socio-historical analysis of the Dutch prison experience*. Edinburgh University Press.

Fraser, A. (2009). Mental health in prisons: A public health agenda. *International Journal of Prisoner Health*, *5*(3), 132–140.

Frechette, J., Bitzas, V., Aubry, M., Kilpatrick, K., & Lavoie-Tremblay, M. (2020). Capturing lived experience: Methodological considerations for interpretive phenomenological inquiry. *International Journal of Qualitative Methods*, *19*. https://doi.org/10.1177/1609406920907254

Freeman, S., & Seymour, M. (2010). 'Just waiting': The nature and effect of uncertainty on young people in remand custody in Ireland. *Youth Justice*, *10*(2), 126–142.

Funnell, S. C., & Rogers, P. J. (2011). *Purposeful program theory: Effective use of theories of change and logic models*. John Wiley & Sons.

Gabriel, Y. (1993). Organizational nostalgia: Reflections on the golden age. In S. Fineman (Ed.), *Emotion in organizations* (pp. 118–141). Sage.

Gadamer, H. G. (2013). *Truth and method*. A&C Black.

Gardner, K. J., Dodsworth, J., & Klonsky, E. D. (2016). Reasons for non-suicidal self-harm in adult male offenders with and without borderline personality traits. *Archives of Suicide Research: Official Journal of the International Academy for Suicide Research*, *20*(4), 614–634.

Garland, D. (1996). The limits of the sovereign states: Strategies of crime control in contemporary society. *British Journal of Criminology*, *36*(4), 445–471.

Garland, D. (1997). Governmentality and the problem of crime: Foucault, criminology, sociology. *Theoretical Criminology*, *1*(2), 173–214.

Garrihy, J., & Watters, A. (2020). Emotions and agency in prison research. *Methodological Innovations*, *13*(2). https://doi.org/10.1177/2059799120926341

Gelsthorpe, L., & Morris, A. (1990). *Feminist perspectives in criminology*. Open University Press.

Giddens, A. (1984). *The constitution of society: Outline of the theory of structuration*. University of California Press.

Gilligan, G., & Pratt, J. (Eds.). (2013). *Crime, truth and justice*. Routledge.

Gladstone, H. (1895). *Report and minutes*. Departmental Committee on Prisons: Gladstone Committee. https://discovery.nationalarchives.gov.uk/details/record?catid=3776982&catln=6

Glaser, B., & Strauss, A. (1967). *The discovery of grounded theory: Strategies for qualitative research*. Sociology Press.

Glesne, C., & Peshkin, A. (1992). *Becoming qualitative researchers*. Longman Publishing Group.

Goffman, E. (1961). *Asylums: Essays on the social situation of mental patients and other inmates'*. Doubleday Anchor.

Good, G. E., Dell, D. M., & Mintz, L. B. (1989). Male role and gender role conflict: Relations to help seeking in men. *Journal of Counseling Psychology*, *36*, 295–300.

Graham, L. (2007). *Prisoner health in Scotland: A healthcare needs assessment*. Scottish Prison Service.

Green, J. D., & Addis, M. E. (2012). Individual differences in masculine gender socialization predictive of men's psychophysiological responses to negative affect. *International Journal of Men's Health*, *11*, 63–82.

Green, J. D., & Jakupcak, M. (2016). Masculinity and men's self-harm behaviors: Implications for non-suicidal self-injury disorder. *Psychology of Men and Masculinity*, *17*(2), 147–155. https://doi.org/10.1037/a0039691

Guiney, T., & Yeomans, H. (2023). Explaining penal momentum: Path dependence, prison population forecasting and the persistence of high incarceration rates in England and Wales. *The Howard Journal of Criminal Justice*, *62*(1), 29–45.

Gupta, B., Iyer, L., & Aronson, J. (2000). Knowledge management: Practices and challenges. *Industrial Management and Data Systems*, *100*(1), 17–21.

Gupta, V., Eames, C., Golding, L., Greenhill, B., Qi, R., Allan, S., Bryant, A., & Fisher, P. (2023). Understanding the identity of lived experience researchers and providers: A conceptual framework and systematic narrative review. *Research Involvement and Engagement*, *9*(1), 26.

Gururajan, V., & Fink, D. (2010). Attitudes towards knowledge transfer in an environment to perform. *Journal of Knowledge Management*. https://doi.org/10.1108/13673271011084880

Hammersley, M. (2015). Research 'inside' viewed from 'outside': Reflections on prison ethnography. In *The Palgrave handbook of prison ethnography* (pp. 21–39). Palgrave Macmillan UK.

Hammersley, M., & Atkinson, P. (1983). *Ethnography: Principles in practice*. Routledge.

Hanlon, M. (2013). Cargo cult science. *European Review*, *21*(1), 51–55.

Hannah-Moffat, K. (2000). Prisons that empower. *British Journal of Criminology*, *40*(3), 510–531.

Harding, C. (1988). 'The inevitable end of a discredited system'? The origins of the Gladstone committee report on prisons, 1895. *The Historical Journal*, *31*(3), 591–608.

Harvey, J. (2007). *Young men in prison: Surviving and adapting to life inside*. Willan Publishing.

Hawton, K., Linsell, L., Adeniji, T., Sariaslan, A., & Fazel, S. (2014). Self-harm in prisons in England and Wales: An epidemiological study of prevalence, risk factors, clustering, and subsequent suicide. *Lancet*, *383*(9923), 1147–1154.

Heath, S., Charles, V., Crow, G., & Wiles, R. (2004). Informed consent, gatekeepers and go-betweens. In *International Association Sixth International Conference on Social Science Methodology*, Amsterdam, August 2004.

Heidegger, M. (1976). *Basic writings from being and time (1927) to the task of thinking (1964)*. Harper and Row.

Heizmann, H., & Olsson, M. R. (2015). Power matters: The importance of Foucault's power/knowledge as a conceptual lens in KM research and practice. *Journal of Knowledge Management*, *19*(4), 756–769.

Hennekam, S. (2019). How to adapt a research design to the particularities of a vulnerable group of workers under study. In *Sage research methods cases part 2*. Sage.

Hinds, L., & Grabosky, P. (2010). Responsibilisation revisited: From concept to attribution in crime control. *Security Journal*, *23*(2), 95–113.

HM Chief Inspector of Prisons for England and Wales (HMCIP). (2007). *The mental health of prisoners: A thematic review of the care and support of prisoners with mental health needs*. The Stationery Office.

HM Chief Inspector of Prisons for England and Wales (HMCIP). (2017). *HM Chief Inspector of Prisons for England and Wales Annual Report 2016–2017*. https://assets.publishing.service.gov.uk/government/uploads/system/uploads/attachment_data/file/629719/hmip-annual-report-2016-17.pdf

HM Chief Inspector of Prisons for England and Wales (HMCIP). (2021). *HM Chief Inspector of Prisons for England and Wales Prison COVID-19 restrictions - Virus suppressed but a heavy toll on prisoners' well-being and rehabilitation*. https://www.justiceinspectorates.gov.uk/hmiprisons/media/pressreleases/2021/02/prison-covid-19-restrictions-virus-suppressed-but-a-heavy-toll-on-prisoners-well-being-and-rehabilitation/

HM Inspectorate of Prisons. (2015). *Life in prison: The first 24 hours in prison*. Her Majesty's Inspectorate of Prisons.

HM Prison Service, Safer Custody Group. (2005). *Prisoner peer support: Good practice guide for insiders peer support schemes*. HMP Safer Custody Group. https://

1library.net/document/yevdr30z-good-practice-guide-for-insiders-peersupport-schemes.html

HMCIP. (2025). The power of an incentivising culture. https://hmiprisons.justiceinspectorates.gov.uk/news/the-power-of-an-incentivising-culture/

HMPPS. (2025). *HM prison & probation service workforce quarterly*. https://www.gov.uk/government/statistics/hm-prison-probation-service-workforce-quarterly-december-2024/hm-prison-and-probation-service-workforce-quarterly-december-2024

Hobhouse, S., & Brockway, F. (1922). *English prisons today*. Prison System Enquiry Committee. https://archive.org/details/englishprisonsto00prisuoft/page/n6/mode/2up

Hockey, J. (2002). Interviews as ethnography? Disembodied social interaction in Britain. In N. Rapport (Ed.), *British subjects: An anthropology of Britain* (pp. 209–222). Berg.

Hockey, J., & Forsey, M. (2012). Ethnography is not participant observation. In J. Skinner (Ed.), *The interview: An ethnographic approach* (pp. 57–75). Berg.

Hollin, C., & Palmer, E. (2006). *Offending behaviour programmes: Development, application and controversies*. John Wiley & Sons.

Holy, L., & Stuchlik, M. (1983). *Actions, norms and representations: Foundations of anthropological enquiry*. Cambridge University Press.

Honeywell, D. (2015). Doing time with lifers: A reflective study of life sentenced prisoners. *British Journal of Community Justice*, *13*(1), 93–104.

House of Commons. (1993). Commons debate. https://publications.parliament.uk/pa/cm199394/cmhansrd/1993-11-23/Debate2.html

Howard League. (2001). *Suicide and self-harm prevention: Court cells and prison vans*. Howard League for Penal Reform.

Ibarra, H., & Obodaru, O. (2016). Betwixt and between identities: Liminal experience in contemporary careers. *Research in Organizational Behavior*, *36*, 47–64.

Illich, I. (1975). Clinical damage, medical monopoly, the expropriation of health: Three dimensions of iatrogenic tort. *Journal of Medical Ethics*, *1*(2), 78–80.

Illich, I. (1976). *Limits to medicine: Medical nemesis - The expropriation of health*. Marion Boyars Publishers.

Ingram, A., Johnson, G., & Heyes, I. (1997). *Self-harm and suicide by detained persons: A study*. Home Office.

Ismail, N. (2020). Rolling back the prison estate: The pervasive impact of macroeconomic austerity on prisoner health in England. *Journal of Public Health*, *42*(3), 625–632.

Ismail, N. (2022). *The English prison health system after a decade of austerity, 2010–2020: The failed political experiment*. Routledge.

Jarrett, C. (2018). Research into the mental health of prisoners, digested. *The British Psychological Society*. https://digest.bps.org.uk/2018/07/13/researchinto-the-mental-health-ofprisoners-digested/

Jewkes, Y. (2005a). Loss, liminality and the life sentence: Managing identity through a disrupted lifecourse. In A. Liebling & S. Maruna (Eds.), *The effects of imprisonment* (pp. 366–388). Willan Publishing.

Jewkes, Y. (2005b). Men behind bars: "Doing" masculinity as an adaptation to imprisonment. *Men and Masculinities*. https://doi.org/10.1177/1097184X03257452

Jewkes, Y. (Ed.). (2007). *Handbook on prisons*. Willan Publishing.

Jewkes, Y. (2012). Autoethnography and emotion as intellectual resources: Doing prison research differently. *Qualitative Inquiry*, *18*(1), 63–75.

Jewkes, Y., & Laws, B. (2021). Liminality revisited: Mapping the emotional adaptations of women in carceral space. *Punishment & Society*, *23*(3), 394–412.

Johnson, R., & McGunigall-Smith, S. (2008). Life without parole, America's other death penalty. *The Prison Journal*, *88*(2), 328–346.

Johnson, R., & Toch, H. (Eds.). (1982). *The pains of imprisonment*. Sage.

Joliffe, D., & Farrington, D. (2007). *A rapid evidence assessment of the impact of mentoring on re-offending*. Home Office.

Jones, H. L. (2007). *The pains of custody: How young men cope through the criminal justice system*. PhD thesis. The University of Hull.

Jupp, V. (1989). *Methods of criminological research*. Routledge.

Kellogg, K. C., Orlikowski, W. J., & Yates, J. A. (2006). Life in the trading zone: Structuring coordination across boundaries in postbureaucratic organizations. *Organization Science*, *17*(1), 22–44.

Kerish, B. R. (1975). Peer counselling. In R. E. Hosford & C. S. Moss (Eds.), *The crumbling walls: Treatment and counselling of offenders*. University of Illinois Press.

Kimmel, M. S. (1994). Masculinity as homophobia: Fear, shame, and silence in the construction of gender identity. In H. Brod & M. Kaufman (Eds.), *Theorizing masculinities* (pp. 119–141). Sage.

Kogut, B., & Zander, U. (1992). Knowledge of the firm, combinative capabilities, and the replication of technology. *Organization Science*, *3*(3), 383–397.

Krumer-Nevo, M., & Benjamin, O. (2010). Critical poverty knowledge: Contesting othering and social distancing. *Current Sociology*, *58*(5), 693–714.

Kupers, A. (2005). Toxic masculinity as a barrier to mental health treatment in prison. *Journal of Clinical Psychology*, *61*(6), 713–724.

Lai, W. (2013). Interoperability of implicit and explicit firm-level knowledge accumulation. *Journal of Strategy and Management*, *6*, 229–241.

Lamb, K., Hegarty, K., Amanda, C. F., & Parker, R. (2020). *The family violence experts by experience framework*. University of Melbourne.

Lazard, L., & McAvoy, J. (2020). Doing reflexivity in psychological research: What's the point? What's the practice? *Qualitative Research in Psychology*, *17*(2), 159–177.

Learmont, J. (1995). *Review of prison service security in England and Wales and the escape from Parkhurst prison on Tuesday 3rd January 1995 (Rep. No. Cm. 3020)*. HMSO.

Leininger, M. (1981). The phenomenon of caring: Importance, research questions and theoretical considerations. In M. Leininger (Ed.), *Caring: An essential human need*. Charles B Slack.

Liamputtong Rice, P., & Ezzy, D. (1999). *Qualitative research methods: A health focus*. Oxford University Press.

Liebling, A. (1992). *Suicides in prison*. Routledge.

Liebling, A. (1995). Vulnerability and prison suicide. *British Journal of Criminology*, *35*(2), 173–187.

Liebling, A. (1999). Prisoner suicide and prisoner coping. *Crime and Justice*, *26*, 283–359.

Liebling, A. (2014). Postscript: Integrity and emotions in prisons research. *Qualitative Inquiry*, *20*(4), 471–486.

Liebling, A. L., Hulley, S., & Crewe, B. (2011). Conceptualising and measuring prison life. In D. Gadd, S. Karstedt, & S. Messner (Eds.), *The Sage handbook of criminological research methods*. Sage.

Liebling, A., & Maruna, S. (2005). *The effects of imprisonment*. Cullompton, Willan.

Lincoln, Y. S., & Denzin, N. K. (1994). The fifth moment. *Handbook of Qualitative Research*, *1*, 575–586.

Lipsky, M. (1969). *Toward a theory of street-level bureaucracy*. Institute for Research on Poverty, University of Wisconsin.

Lipton, D. S., Martinson, R., & Wilks, J. (1975). *The effectiveness of correctional treatment: A survey of treatment evaluation studies*. Praeger.

Lloyd, C. (1990). *Suicide and self-injury in prison: A literature review* (Vol. 115). HM Stationery Office.

Lo, J. (2019). Exploring the buffer effect of receiving social support on lonely and emotionally unstable social networking users. *Computers in Human Behavior*, *90*, 103–116.

Lofland, J., & Lofland, L. H. (1995). Developing analysis. In J. Lofland, D. A. Snow, L. Anderson, & L. H. Lofland (Eds.), *Analyzing social settings: A guide to qualitative observation and analysis* (pp. 183–203). Waveland Press.

Lohner, J., & Konrad, N. (2007). Risk factors for self-injurious behaviour in custody: Problems of definition and prediction. *International Journal of Prisoner Health*, *3*(2), 135–161.

Lukes, S. (2005). Power and the battle for hearts and minds. *Millennium*, *33*(3), 477–493.

Maden, M., Cunliffe, A., McMahon, N., Booth, A., Carey, G. M., Paisley, S., Dickson, R., & Gabbay, M. (2017). Use of programme theory to understand the differential effects of interventions across socio-economic groups in systematic reviews—A systematic methodology review. *Systematic Reviews*, *6*(1), 1–23.

Magnier-Watanabe, R. (2011). Getting ready for kaizen: Organizational and knowledge management enablers. *Vine*, *41*(4), 428–448.

Marder, I., Lapouge, M., Garrihy, J., & Brandon, A. (2021). Empirical research on the impact and experience of open prisons: State of the field and future directions. *Prison Service Journal*, *256*, 3–9.

Marouf, L. N. (2007). Social networks and knowledge sharing in organizations: A case study. *Journal of Knowledge Management*, *11*(6), 110–125.

Marshall, N. (2006). Understanding power in project settings. In D. Hodgson & S. Cicmil (Eds.), *Making projects critical* (pp. 207–231). Palgrave Macmillan.

Martel, J. (2004). Policing criminological knowledge: The hazards of qualitative research on women in prison. *Theoretical Criminology*, *8*(2), 157–189.

Maruna, S. (2011a). Reentry as a rite of passage. *Punishment & Society*, *13*(1), 3–28.

Maruna, S. (2011b). Why do they hate us? Making peace between prisoners and psychology. *International Journal of Offender Therapy and Comparative Criminology*, *55*(5), 671–675.

Maruna, S., McNaull, G., & O'Neill, N. (2022). The COVID-19 pandemic and the future of the prison. *Crime and Justice*, *51*(1), 59–103.

Mathie, E., & Ford, N. (1998). Peer education for health. In K. Topping & S. Ehly (Eds.), *Peer-assisted learning* (pp. 203–218). Routledge.

Matthews, R. (2005). The myth of punitiveness. *Theoretical Criminology*, *9*(2), 175–201.

Matthews, R. (2014). *Realist criminology*. Palgrave Macmillan.

Mayhew, H. (1862). *The criminal prisons of London and scenes of prison life*. Griffin, Bohn, and Company.

McCord, J. (2003). Cures that harm: Unanticipated outcomes of crime prevention programs. *The Annals of the American Academy of Political and Social Science*, *587*(1), 16–30.

McFadyen, J., & Rankin, J. (2016). The role of gatekeepers in research: Learning from reflexivity and reflection. *GSTF Journal of Nursing and Health Care*, *4*(1), 82–88.

McGarry, O. (2016). Repositioning the research encounter: Exploring power dynamics and positionality in youth research. *International Journal of Social Research Methodology*, *19*(3), 339–354.

McHugh, M. (1995). Managing suicidal behaviour among the prison population. *Perspectives in Public Health*, *115*(2). https://doi.org/10.1177/146642409511500211

McKinnon, J. L., Harrison, G. L., Chow, C. W., & Wu, A. (2003). Organizational culture: Association with commitment, job satisfaction, propensity to remain, and information sharing in Taiwan. *International Journal of Business Studies*, *11*(1), 25–44.

McLeod, K. E., Butler, A., Young, J. T., Southalan, L., Borschmann, R., Sturup-Toft, S., Dirkzwager, A., Dolan, K., Acheampong, L. K., Topp, S. M., & Martin, R. E. (2020). Global prison health care governance and health equity: A critical lack of evidence. *American Journal of Public Health*, *110*(3), 303–308.

McMahon, M. (1992). *The persistent prison? Rethinking decarceration and penal reform*. University of Toronto Press.

McNichols, D. (2010). Optimal knowledge transfer methods: A generation X perspective. *Journal of Knowledge Management*, *14*(1), 24–37.

Mead, G. H. (1934). *Mind, self, and society from the standpoint of a social behaviorist*. University of Chicago Press.

Mears, D. P. (2007). Towards rational and evidence-based crime policy. *Journal of Criminal Justice*, *35*(6), 667–682.

Mertens, D. M., & Wilson, A. (2012). *Program evaluation: Theory and practice*. Guilford Press.

Merton, R. K. (1972). Insiders and outsiders: A chapter in the sociology of knowledge. *American Journal of Sociology*, *78*(1), 9–47.

Meško, G., & Hacin, R. (2018). Prisoners' and prison workers' views on the prison subculture in Slovenia. *Revija za Kriminalistiko in Kriminologijo/Ljubljana*, *69*(4), 333–345.

Mesmer-Magnus, J., & DeChurch, L. (2009). Information sharing and team performance: A meta-analysis. *Journal of Applied Psychology*, *94*(2), 535–546.

Milburn, K. (1995). A critical review of peer education with young people with special reference to sexual health. *Health Education Research*, *10*(4), 407–420.

Miličević, A., Simić, M., Bogdanović, Z., Despotović-Zrakić, M., & Suvajdžić, M. (2025, February). Entrepreneurship education approaches: Hackathon and project-based learning. In *Entrepreneurship education in central and East Europe* (pp. 83–111). Nomos Verlagsgesellschaft mbH & Co. KG.

Miller, W., & MacGilchrist, L. (1996). A model for peer-led work. *Health Education*, *96*(2), 24–29.

Ministry of Justice. (2020). *Areas of research interest*. https://assets.publishing.service.gov.uk/government/uploads/system/uploads/attachment_data/file/1007378/areas-of-research-interest.pdf

Ministry of Justice. (2022). *Prison population figures: 2022*. https://www.gov.uk/government/publications/prison-population-figures-2022

Ministry of Justice. (2025a). *Prisons data*. https://data.justice.gov.uk/prisons

Ministry of Justice. (2025b). *Prisons data*. https://data.justice.gov.uk/prisons

Ministry of Justice. (2025c). *Safer in custody: Quarterly update to September 2024*. https://www.gov.uk/government/statistics/safety-in-custody-quarterly-update-to-september-2024

Ministry of Justice. (n.d.). *Prison security categories*. https://www.gov.uk/life-in-prison/prison-security-categories

Mjåland, K., Laursen, J., Schliehe, A., & Larmour, S. (2023). Contrasts in freedom: Comparing the experiences of imprisonment in open and closed prisons in England and Wales and Norway. *European Journal of Criminology*, *20*(5), 1641–1662.

Moran, D. (2013). Between outside and inside? Prison visiting rooms as liminal carceral spaces. *Geojournal*, *78*, 339–351. https://doi.org/10.1007/s10708-011-9442-6

Morris, T., & Morris, P. (1963). *Pentonville: A sociological study of an English prison* (1st ed.). Routledge. https://doi.org/10.4324/9781315007915

Nakano, D., Muniz, J., & Batista, E. D. (2013). Engaging environments: Tacit knowledge sharing on the shop floor. *Journal of Knowledge Management*, *17*(2), 290–306.

Nam, S. K., Chu, H., Lee, M., Lee, J., Kim, N., & Lee, S. (2010). A Meta-analysis of gender differences in attitudes toward seeking professional psychological help. *Journal of American College Health*, *59*(2), 110–116.

National Audit Office. (2010). *Managing offenders on short custodial sentences*. National Audit Office.

National Audit Office. (2017). *Mental health in prisons*. https://www.nao.org.uk/wp-content/uploads/2017/06/Mental-health-in-prisons.pdf

National Offender Management Service (NOMS). (2015). *Early days in custody – Reception in, first night in custody, and induction to custody*. https://assets.publishing.service.gov.uk/government/uploads/system/uploads/attachment_data/file/889890/psi-07-2015-pi-06-2015-early-days-custody.pdf

Nelson, L. J. (n.d.). *Congratulations: You have survived the war. Now live with the trauma* [Quote]. Goodreads. https://goodreads.com/quotes

Nonaka, I., & Takeuchi, H. (1995). *The knowledge-creating company: How Japanese companies create the dynamics of innovation*. Oxford University Press.

O'Malley, P. A. T. (1999). Volatile and contradictory punishment. *Theoretical Criminology*, *3*(2), 175–196.

Palinkas, L. A., Horwitz, S. M., Green, C. A., Wisdom, J. P., Duan, N., & Hoagwood, K. (2015, September). Purposeful sampling for qualitative data collection and analysis in mixed method implementation research. *Administration and Policy in Mental Health and Mental Health Services Research*, *42*(5), 533–544. https://doi.org/10.1007/s10488-013-0528-y

Parisi, N. (1982). The prisoner's pressures and responses. In N. Parisi (Ed.), *Coping with imprisonment* (pp. 9–26). Sage.

Parkin, S., & McKeganey, N. (2000). The rise and rise of peer education approaches. *Drugs: Education, Prevention & Policy*, *7*(3), 293–310.

Parsons, C., Maras, P., Knowles, C., Bradshaw, V., Hollingworth, K., & Monteiro, H. (2008). *Formalised peer mentoring pilot evaluation*. http://webarchive.national

archives.gov.uk/20130401151715/http://www.education.gov.uk/publications/eorderingdownload/dcsf-rr033-r.pdf

Paulus, P., & Dzindolet, M. (1992). The effects of prison confinement. In P. Suedfeld & P. Tetlock (Eds.), *Psychology and social policy* (pp. 327–341). Hemisphere Publishing.

Peay, J. (2017). Mental health, mental disabilities and crime. In A. Liebling, S. Maruna, & L. McAra (Eds.), *The Oxford handbook of criminology*. Oxford University Press.

Penal Reform International. (2022). *Global prison trends 2022*. https://cdn.penalreform.org/wp-content/uploads/2022/05/GPT2022.pdf

Perrin, C. (2017). *The untapped utility of peer-support programs in prisons and implications for theory, policy, and practice*. PhD Thesis. Nottingham Trent University.

Perrin, C. (2019). Peer support and individuals with sexual convictions: Complementing traditional rehabilitation strategies. In *Sexual crime and the experience of imprisonment* (pp. 143–169). Palgrave Macmillan.

Perrin, C. (2024). *Peer support in prison: How incarcerated people make meaning through active citizenship*. Taylor & Francis.

Phillips, C., & Earle, R. (2010). Reading difference differently? Identity, epistemology and prison ethnography. *British Journal of Criminology*, *50*(2), 360–378.

Player, E., & Jenkins, M. (1994). *Prisons after Woolf*. Routledge.

Pollitt, C. (1993). *Managerialism and the public services: Cuts or cultural change in the 1990s?* Blackwell.

Potter, H. (2019). *Shades of the prison house: A history of incarceration in the British Isles*. Boydell and Brewer.

Poulin, F., Dishion, T. J., & Burraston, B. (2001). 3-year iatrogenic effects associated with aggregating high-risk adolescents in cognitive-behavioral preventive interventions. *Applied Developmental Science*, *5*(4), 214–224.

Pratt, J., Brown, D., Brown, M., Hallsworth, S., & Morrison, W. (Eds.). (2005). *The new punitiveness: Trends, theories, perspectives*. Willan Publishing.

Prison Guide. (2022). *Category D open prison*. https://prisonguide.co.uk/category-d-open-prison/

Prison Reform Trust. (1991). The Woolf report: A summary of the main findings and recommendations of the inquiry into prison disturbances. https://prisonreformtrust.org.uk/publication/the-woolf-report-a-summary-of-themain-findings-and-recommendations-of-the-inquiry-into-prison-disturbances

Prison Reform Trust. (2019a). Bromley briefings summer 2019. https://prisonreformtrust.org.uk/wpcontent/uploads/old_files/Documents/Bromley%20Briefings/Prison%20the%20facts%20Summer%202019.pdf

Prison Reform Trust. (2019b, August 20). Release on temporary licence (ROTL). https://prisonreformtrust.org.uk/release-on-temporary-licence-rotl/

Reed, J. (1992). *Review of health and social services for mentally disordered offenders and others requiring similar services: Presented to parliament by the secretary of state for health and the home department (Cm 2088)*. The Stationery Office.

Rhule, D. M. (2005). Take care to do no harm: Harmful interventions for youth problem behavior. *Professional Psychology: Research and Practice*, *36*(6), 618.

Richards, S. C., & Ross, J. I. (2001). Introducing the new school of convict criminology. *Social Justice*, *28*(1), 177–190.

Rivera-Vazquez, J. C., Ortiz-Fournier, L. V., & Flores, F. R. (2009). Overcoming cultural barriers for innovation and knowledge sharing. *Journal of Knowledge Management*, *13*(5), 257–270.

Rogers, P. J., Petrosino, A., Huebner, T. A., & Hacsi, T. A. (2000). Program theory evaluation: Practice, promise, and problems. *New Directions for Evaluation*, *87*, 5–13.

Rose, N. (1996). Governing "advanced" liberal democracies. In A. Sharma & A. Gupta (Eds.), *The anthropology of the state: A reader*. Blackwell.

Rose, N. (2000). Government and control. *British Journal of Criminology*, *40*(2), 321–339.

Rossi, P. H., Lipsey, M. W., & Freeman, H. E. (2004). *Evaluation: A systematic approach* (7th ed.). Sage.

Rowe, A. (2015). Situating the self in prison research: Power, identity and epistemology. In D. H. Drake, R. Earle, & J. Sloan (Eds.), *The Palgrave handbook of prison ethnography. Palgrave studies in prisons and penology*. Palgrave Macmillan. https://doi.org/10.1057/9781137403889_19

Ryan, L. (2015). Inside and Outside of what or where? Researching migration through multi-positionalities. *Forum qualitative Social Research*, *16*.

Ryan, T. A., & McCabe, K. A. (1994). Mandatory versus voluntary prison education and academic achievement. *The Prison Journal*, *74*(4), 450–461.

Sanghera, G. S., & Thapar-Bjorkert, S. (2008). Methodological dilemmas: Gatekeepers and positionality in Bradford. *Ethnic and Racial Studies*, *31*(3), 543–562.

Sapsford, R. (1983). *Life sentence prisoners: Reaction, response and change*. Open University Press.

Savin-Baden, M., & Major, C. (2013). *Qualitative research: The essential guide to theory and practice*. Routledge.

Savolainen, J., Casey, P. J., McBrayer, J. P., & Schwerdtle, P. N. (2023). Positionality and its problems: Questioning the value of reflexivity statements in research. *Perspectives on Psychological Science*, *18*(6), 1331–1338.

Schreeche-Powell, E. (2019). Becoming me with The Open University. In R. Earle & J. Mehigan (Eds.), *Degrees of freedom: Prison education and The Open University* (pp. 165–176). Policy Press/Bristol University Press.

Schreeche-Powell, E. (2020). Peer support and well-being: Exploring the impact of peer-led induction on male prisoners. *Journal of Prisoners on Prisons*, *29*(1–2), 30–60.

Schreeche-Powell, E. (2023). *Peer support in prisons: Exploring the role and experience of peer-led induction on male prisoners in their transfer and transition to open prison*. Doctoral dissertation. University of Kent, N/A.

Schreeche-Powell, E. (2025). Insecurity and fragility: The perpetual duo of precarity for 'convict criminologists' in a risk averse academy. *Critical Criminology*, 1–16.

Scott, D. (2006). The caretakers of punishment: Prison officer personal authority and the rule of law. *Prison Service Journal*, *168*, 14–19.

Scott, D. (2016). Iatrogenic harm in prison. In K. Corteen, S. Morley, P. Taylor, & J. Turner (Eds.), *A companion to crime, harm and victimisation*. Policy Press.

Scott, D., & Codd, H. (2010). *Controversial issues in prisons*. Open University Press.

Scott, D., Harzke, A. J., Mizwa, M. B., Pugh, M., & Ross, M. W. (2004). Evaluation of an HIV peer education program in Texas prisons. *Journal of Corrective Health, 10*(2), 151–173.

Scowcroft, E., Slade, K., Winder, B., & Oldfield, B. (2019). *Exploring the effectiveness of Samaritans' Listener Scheme and prisoner suicide through the lens of the IMV model of suicidal behaviour*. Doctoral dissertation. Nottingham Trent University.

Sedenu, A. (2005). Safer custody group. *The British Journal of Forensic Practice, 7*(4), 14–20. https://doi.org/10.1108/14636646200500024

Shaghaghi, A., Bhopal, R. S., & Sheikh, A. (2011). Approaches to recruiting 'hard-to-reach' populations into research: A review of the literature. *Health Promotion Perspectives, 1*(2), 86–94.

Shamir, R. (2008). The age of responsibilization: On market-embedded morality. *Economy and Society, 37*(1), 1–19.

Shammas, V. L. (2014). The pains of freedom: Assessing the ambiguity of Scandinavian penal exceptionalism on Norway's Prison Island. *Punishment & Society, 16*(1), 104–123.

Shammas, V. L. (2017). *Pains of imprisonment. Encyclopaedia of corrections*. Wiley-Blackwell.

Shaw, D. (2019, June 4). Offender rehabilitation schemes 'not tested'. *The BBC*. https://www.bbc.co.uk/news/uk-48516286

Shiner, M. (1999). Defining peer education. *Journal of Adolescence, 22*(4), 555–566.

Simmel, G. (1950). *The sociology of Georg Simmel* (Translated from German by Kurt H. Wolff). The Free Press.

Singleton, N., Bumpstead, R., O'Brien, N., Lee, A., & Meltzer, H. (2001). *Psychiatric morbidity among adults living in private households, 2000*. Office of National Statistics, HMSO.

Singleton, N., Meltzer, H., & Gatward, R. (1998). *Psychiatric morbidity among prisoners in England and Wales*. Office for National Statistics.

Siu, H. (n.d.). *It is a lot better to walk alone than with a crowd going in the wrong direction* [Quote]. https://goodreads.com/quotes

Snow, L., & Biggar, K. (2006). The role of peer support in reducing self-harm in prisons. In G. E. Dear (Ed.), *Preventing suicide and other self-harm in prison* (pp. 153–166). Palgrave.

South, J., Bagnall, A., Hulme, C., Woodall, J., Longo, R., Dixey, R., Kinsella, K., Raine, G., Vinall, K., & Wright, J. (2014). *A systematic review of the effectiveness and cost-effectiveness of peer-based interventions to maintain and improve offender health in prison settings*. NIHR Journals Library.

Spierenburg, P. (2004). Punishment, power, and history: Foucault and Elias. *Social Science History, 28*(4), 607–636.

Spurr, M., & Bennett, J. (2008). The interview: Michael Spurr. *Prison Service Journal, 177*, 54–61.

Statham, B. M., Winder, B., & Micklethwaite, D. (2021). Success within a UK open prison and surviving the 'pains of freedom'. *Psychology, Crime and Law, 27*(8), 729–750.

Stearns, P. (1979). *Be a man! Males in modern society*. Holmes & Meier Publishers.

Stevens, A., Schreeche-Powell, E., Billingham, L., & Irwin-Rogers, K. (2025). Interventionitis in the criminal justice system: Three English cases. *Critical Criminology*, 1–17.

Stewart, D. (2008). *The problems and needs of newly sentenced prisoners: Results from a national survey*. Ministry of Justice.

Sturup-Toft, S., O'Moore, E. J., & Plugge, E. H. (2018). Looking behind the bars: Emerging health issues for people in prison. *British Medical Bulletin, 125*, 15–23. https://doi.org/10.1093/bmb/ldx052

Suchman, E. A. (1967). *Evaluative research: Principles and practice in public service and social action programs*. Russell Sage Foundation.

Sykes, G. (1958). *The society of captives: A study of a maximum-security prison*. Princeton University Press.

Taylor, C. (2021, May 14). Chief Inspector's blog: Open prisons in lockdown [Blog post]. *HM Inspectorate of Prisons*. https://www.justiceinspectorates.gov.uk/hmiprisons/chief-inspectors-blog/chiefinspectors-blog-open-prisons-lockdown

The Guardian. (2013, May 24). Unthinkable? Hooray for tick-box culture. [Editorial]. *The Guardian*. [online] https://www.theguardian.com/commentisfree/2013/may/24/unthinkable-box-ticking-approval

The Joint Committee on Human Rights. (2004). *Deaths in custody: Third report of session 2004–05* (Vol. 1). The Stationery Office.

The Samaritans. (2022). The listener scheme. https://www.samaritans.org/how-we-can-help/prisons/listener-scheme

Tolan, P., Henry, D., Schoeny, M., Bass, A., Lovegorve, P., & Nichols, E. (2008). Mentoring interventions to affect juvenile delinquency and associated problems: A systemic review. *Campbell Systemic Reviews*, *9*(1), 1–158.

Torfing, J. (2013). Power and discourse: Towards an anti-foundationalist concept of power. In S. R. Clegg & M. Haugaard (Eds.), *The SAGE handbook of power* (pp. 108–124). SAGE.

Townley, B. (1993). Foucault, power/knowledge, and its relevance for human resource management. *Academy of Management Review*, *18*(3), 518–545.

Tubex, H. (2015). Reach and relevance of prison research. *International Journal for Crime, Justice and Social Democracy*, *4*(1), 4–17. https://doi.org/10.5204/ijcjsd.v4i1.200

Turner, V. (1967). *The forest of symbols: Aspects of ndembu ritual*. Cornell University Press.

Turner, G., & Shepherd, J. (1999). A method in search of a theory: Peer education and health promotion. *Health Education Research*, *14*(2), 235–247.

Uzkurt, C., Kumar, R., Kimzan, H., & Eminoglu, G. (2013). Role of innovation in the relationship between organizational culture and firm performance. *European Journal of Innovation Management*, *16*, 92–117.

Van Gennep, A. (1909). *Les Rites de passage*. A. et J. Picard.

Van Gennep, A. (1960). *The rites of passage*. Routledge and Kegan Paul.

Von Meier, A. (1999). Occupational cultures as a challenge to technological innovation. *IEEE Transactions on Engineering Management*, *46*(1), 101–114.

Walker, S., & Avis, M. (1999). Common reasons why peer education fails. *Journal of Adolescence*, *22*, 573–577.

Walkerdine, V., Lucey, H., & Melody, J. (2012). Growing up girl: Psychosocial explorations of gender and class. In *Off white* (pp. 98–113). Routledge.

Walton, H., Massou, E., Sherlaw-Johnson, C., Gipson, D., Wainwright, L., & Harriott, P. (2025). Peer support for adult social care in prisons in England and

Wales: A mixed-methods rapid evaluation. *Health and Social Care Delivery Research*, *13*(01). https://doi.org/10.3310/MWFD6890

Walton, H., Tomini, S. M., Sherlaw-Johnson, C., Ng, P. L., & Fulop, N. J. (2023). How is social care provided in adult prisons in England and Wales? *British Journal of Social Work*, *53*, 718–736.

Weinrath, M. (2016). *Behind the Walls: Inmates and correctional officers on the State of Canadian prisons*. UBC Press.

Wels, H., Van der Waal, K., Spiegel, A., & Kamsteeg, F. (2011). Victor Turner and liminality: An introduction. *Anthropology Southern Africa*, *34*(1–2), 1–4.

Welsh, B. C., & Rocque, M. (2014). When crime prevention harms: A review of systematic reviews. *Journal of Experimental Criminology*, *10*(3), 245–266.

Whitlock, J., Muehlenkamp, J., Purington, A., Eckenrode, J., Barreira, P., Baral Abrams, G., Marchell, T., Kress, V., Girard, K., Chin, C., & Knox, K. (2011). Nonsuicidal self-injury in a college population: General trends and sex differences. *Journal of American College Health*, *59*(8), 691–698.

Winslade, J. M. (2005). Utilising discursive positioning in counselling. *British Journal of Guidance and Counselling*, *33*(3), 351–364.

Wolcott, H. (1990). *Writing up qualitative research*. Sage.

Woodall, J., South, J., Dixey, R., De Viggiani, N., & Penson, B. (2015). Expert views of peer-based interventions for prisoner health. *International Journal of Prisoner Health*, *11*(2), 87–97.

Woolf, H., & Tumin, S. (1991). *Prison disturbances April 1990: Report of an inquiry (Cm 1456)*. HMSO.

World Health Organisation. (1998). *Mental health promotion in prisons: Report on a WHO meeting*. http://www.euro.who.int/__data/assets/pdf_file/0007/99016/E64328.pdf

Wrong, D. H. (2017). *Power: Its forms, bases, and uses*. Routledge.

Yuen, F. (2011). "I've never been so free in all my life": Healing through aboriginal ceremonies in prison. *Leisure/Loisir*, *35*(2), 97–113.

Zane, S. N., Welsh, B. C., & Zimmerman, G. M. (2016). Examining the iatrogenic effects of the Cambridge-Somerville youth study: Existing explanations and new appraisals. *British Journal of Criminology*, *56*(1), 141–160.

Zboralski, K. (2009). Antecedents of knowledge sharing in communities of practice. *Journal of Knowledge Management*, *13*, 90–101.

Zietsma, C., & Lawrence, T. B. (2010). Institutional work in the transformation of an organizational field: The interplay of boundary work and practice work. *Administrative Science Quarterly*, *55*(2), 189–221.

Index

Printed and bound by CPI Group (UK) Ltd, Croydon, CR0 4YY

01/06/2026

14890759-0001